Great Medical Disasters

Great Medical Disasters

RICHARD GORDON

Hutchinson

London Melbourne Sydney Auckland Johannesburg

Hutchinson & Co. (Publishers) Ltd

An imprint of the Hutchinson Publishing Group

17–21 Conway Street, London W1P 6JD

Hutchinson Group (Australia) Pty Ltd
30–32 Cremorne Street, Richmond South, Victoria 3121
PO Box 151, Broadway, New South Wales 2007

Hutchinson Group (NZ) Ltd
32–34 View Road, PO Box 40–086, Glenfield, Auckland 10

Hutchinson Group (SA) Pty Ltd
PO Box 337, Bergvlei 2012, South Africa

First published 1983
© Richard Gordon Limited 1983

Set in Linotron Baskerville by Input Typesetting Ltd, London SW19 8DR

Printed in Great Britain by The Anchor Press Ltd
and bound by Wm Brendon & Son Ltd,
both of Tiptree, Essex

British Library Cataloguing in Publication Data

Gordon, Richard
    Great medical disasters.
    1. Medicine–Anecdotes, facetiae, satire, etc.
    I. Title
    610   R705

ISBN 0 09 152230 7

Physicians of all men are most happy; what good success soever they have, the world proclaimeth, and what faults they commit, the earth coverest.

FRANCIS QUARLES

Doctors pour drugs of which they know little, to cure diseases of which they know less, into human beings of whom they know nothing.

VOLTAIRE

The medical profession has not a high character; it has an infamous character.

BERNARD SHAW

Medicine is a rather philistine sort of profession; it's so often used to acquire rank and status. So many people are attracted to medicine because it will guarantee they will always be respected and important to society.

DR JONATHAN MILLER

The medical is an invidious profession. When one's practice is among the rich one looks like a lackey, when it's among the poor like a thief.

DR LOUIS-FERDINAND CÉLINE

Medicine is an art founded on conjecture and improved by murder.

SIR ANTHONY CARLISLE

See one physician like a sculler plies
The patient lingers and by inches dies.
But two physicians like a pair of oars
Waft him more swiftly to the Stygian shores.

ANON

He that sinneth before his Maker, let him fall
into the hand of the physician.

ECCLESIASTICUS, 28:15

Doctors are professional and graduated homicides.

SYDNEY SMITH

Doctors is all swabs.

BILLY BONES in *Treasure Island*

Contents

Contents

Contents

A Disastrous Practice

Thousands of books have been published on the triumphs of medicine.

This is the other one.

Medicine has its Tay Bridge, *Titanic*, Great Fire of London and San Francisco Earthquake.

Even its equivalents of pussies up trees, burst water-mains and thunderstorms are major disasters if they happen to *you*.

Mankind suffered cruelly for centuries from lack of medical knowledge. The brilliant scientific discoveries of our own century eradicated the evil so efficiently it now suffers as painfully from too much.

Doctors can be fired by ideals – as fanatically as the Spanish Inquisition. They can follow more false trails than Inspector Clouseau. They can become so fond of dead doctrines that medical progress resembles a procession of ostriches with their heads in the sand.

The medical art is more revealed by its disasters, as the military one by its defeats.

This catalogue of disasters will make you feel great to be alive.

1

Triple Knock-Out
Disastrous surgical enthusiasm

Robert Liston was the fastest knife in the West End. He could amputate a leg in 2½ minutes.

He lived during the 1840s at No. 5 Clifford Street, off Bond Street in Mayfair. His three-storey house with tall downstairs windows, elegantly spiralling oak staircase and boot-scraper, now faces the club which invented Buck's fizz.

Liston was an incorrigible bustler, even for a surgeon. He eschewed carriages, visited his patients on horseback and loved hunting. His reputation for speedy wizardry so choked his waiting room, the butler had to circulate a reviving decanter of madeira and biscuits. Then anaesthesia was unknown – you had the choice of fuddling with opium or rum, or biting on a cloth-wrapped peg – and surgery was a matter of more haste, less pain.

He was six foot two, and operated in a bottle-green coat with wellington boots. He sprung across the blood-stained boards upon his swooning, sweating, strapped-down patient like a duellist, calling, 'Time me, gentlemen, time me!' to students craning with pocket watches from the iron-railinged galleries. Everyone swore that the first flash of his knife was followed so swiftly by the rasp of saw on bone that sight and sound seemed simultaneous. To free both hands, he would clasp the bloody knife between his teeth.

Liston invented see-through isinglass sticking plaster, the 'bulldog' artery forceps, and a leg splint still used during World War Two. The son of a Scots minister, he graduated from Edinburgh, became first 'The Great North-

13

ern Anatomist' of *Blackwood's Magazine*, and was rumoured enthusiastically to 'resurrect' his own corpses.

An abrupt, abrasive, argumentative man, unfailingly charitable to the poor and tender to the sick, impossibly vain, he was vilely unpopular among his fellow surgeons at the Edinburgh Royal Infirmary. He relished operating successfully in the reeking tenements of the Grassmarket and Lawnmarket on patients they had discharged as hopelessly incurable. They conspired to bar him from the wards, banished him south, where he became professor of surgery at University College Hospital in London and made a fortune.

It was Robert Liston who performed on 21 December 1846 the first operation under anaesthesia in Europe. His only comment – 'This Yankee dodge beats mesmerism hollow.' The leg hit the sawdust in the bucket after 2½ minutes, but his talent for surgical velocity was already outdated.

Liston's fourth most famous case

Removal in 4 minutes of a 45-pound scrotal tumour, whose owner had to carry it round in a wheelbarrow.

Liston's third most famous case

Argument with his house-surgeon. Was the red, pulsating tumour in a small boy's neck a straightforward abscess of the skin? Or a dangerous aneurism of the carotid artery?

'Pooh!' Liston exclaimed impatiently. 'Whoever heard of an aneurism in a boy so young?' Flashing a knife from his waistcoat pocket, he lanced it. Houseman's note – 'Out leaped arterial blood, and the boy fell.' The patient died but the artery lives, in University College Hospital pathology museum, specimen No. 1256.

Liston's second most famous case

Amputated the leg in 2½ minutes, but in his enthusiasm the patient's testicles as well.

Liston's most famous case

Amputated the leg *under* 2½ minutes (the patient died afterwards in the ward from hospital gangrene, they usually did in those pre-Listerian days). He amputated in addition the fingers of his young assistant (who died afterwards in the ward from hospital gangrene, they usually did in those pre-Listerian days). He also slashed through the coat tails of a distinguished surgical spectator, who was so terrified that the knife had pierced his vitals he dropped dead from fright.

That was the only operation in history with a 300 per cent mortality.

2

Untreasured Island

How to beat Hitler with sheep

'We shall fight on the beaches,' Winston Churchill challenged during the disastrous Dunkirk week of June 1940. 'We shall fight on the landing grounds, we shall fight in the fields and in the streets, we shall fight in the hills.'

He might have added, 'And on a small island off the northwest coast of Scotland, with rather more chance of success.'

Hitler and his friends were in charge from Tokyo Bay to Algeciras Bay, from Murmansk to Mersa Matrûh. There was nothing that lovely summer to stop him shooting the bluebirds and landing on the White Cliffs of Dover.

We British set about defending our precious stone set in a silver sea with customary endearing crankiness. All signposts were removed, so Nazi parachutists, invariably dressed as nuns, would betray themselves at rustic crossroads with paroxisms of Teutonic choler over the correct route from Husbands Bosworth to Husborne Crawley, or if in Wales from Llansantffraid Glyn-Ceirog to Llansantff-aid yn Mechain.

The fields were scattered with oil drums, spiky harrows, rusty potato-planters and broken-down tractors, scarecrows against more Nazi nuns arriving by glider. The shore was unwelcoming with prickly lengths of railway line. British housewives beat their aluminium saucepans into Spitfires. Nothing was too devilish for Hitler.

Dr Paul Fildes, of the Chemical Defence Experimental Establishment, gazed through his laboratory window across the lovely Wiltshire countryside of Porton Down, and dreamed of anthrax.

The *Bacillus anthracis* is a microbial giant, a square-ended rod generally going about in pairs. On nutrient jelly it grows greyish felt-like blobs, with tangled edges microscopically resembling curly hair – the 'Medusa head'. One glance from Gorgon Medusa instantly turned you to stone, one touch from the anthrax bacillus could be equally calamitous.

There are two sorts of anthrax. One from an infected scratch, a black scab surrounded by bursting blebs of skin, with the trivial mortality of 25 per cent. And anthrax of the lungs, 'woolsorters' disease', described in a 1940 textbook of medicine with gusto – 'Onset rapid. Rigor, rapid respiration, pain in chest, rapid and feeble pulse. Cough and bronchitis usual. *Temperature high.* Oedema of chest wall develops, of gelatinous consistency. Much frothy mucus. Extreme collapse and death in one to three days.'

Exactly what any Englishman would then have wished any German, particularly as the account ends, 'Mind usually remains clear.'

Anthrax was a disease of farmers and vets and men working in slaughterhouses. No one had thought of it as a weapon of war before. The difficulty was extending these startling effects to the entire population of the Ruhr. Dr Fildes knew you sometimes got it from shaving brushes, but this did not seem enormously useful, apart from humanely sparing the women and children.

16

It was no problem in a summer of desperate resourcefulness, when old ladies learned to mix (later-named) Molotov cocktails, when the rifleless Home Guard commandeered pitchforks to stick into the descending buttocks of parachuting nuns. The RAF diverted briefly from the Battle of Britain to design anthrax bomblets.

These bomblets would be packed with billions of anthrax spores, disseminated with a small, economical charge. A recommendation for bombarding the Germans with anthrax rather than, say, *Pasteurella pestis* of the Black Death, was this handy ability of each microbe to armour itself with a thick spore. Once again in a warm, moist, airy environment with its customary nutrients, the spore became its old self and ready to fight for King and country.

The next task was trying out the secret weapon. The Army's traditional testing ground of Salisbury Plain carried the disadvantage of possibly wiping out the inhabitants of Salisbury. So many unlikely corners of the British Isles were already commandeered for military use – divers jostled with the Monster in Loch Ness, St James's Park opposite Buckingham Palace was full of anti-aircraft balloons, Brighton front was thick with pillboxes camouflaged as ice-cream kiosks.

The War Office swooped on Gruinard Island. It was a mile long and half a mile wide. It stood a couple of miles offshore in hilly Gruinard Bay, which looked northeast from the convoluted Wester Ross coast across the North Minch towards Stornoway in the Outer Hebrides. Better still, it was uninhabited.

In the spring of 1941, when London, Coventry and elsewhere had been ravaged by the Luftwaffe, when Roosevelt had pushed Lend-Lease through Congress, when Hitler was contemplating invading Russia, and when his Deputy Führer was contemplating dropping into the Duke of Hamilton from his Messerschmitt 150 miles to the south, Dr Fildes was ready at Gruinard Island.

He arrived with several army lorries full of sheep. Sixty hapless baaing contributors to the war effort were ferried across the bay, tethered to stakes scattered over the rock-strewn Gruinard grass beneath gantries of poles and planks, and showered with anthrax spores from exploded bomblets. The experiment was successful beyond its engineer's dreams. Every sheep was shortly dead.

The rest was pencil-and-paper work.

Anthrax was clearly more effective than TNT. The British before the Blitz awarded each ton of Nazi bombs a 'multiplier' of 50, meaning fifty civilian casualties. (This was flattering to the Luftwaffe, which in the Spanish Civil War achieved a multiplier of only 17.2.) The inhabitants of Berlin, Frankfurt, Stuttgart and Hamburg were generously given 50 per cent of the ovine death rate on Gruinard. A hundred bomblets clustered in a 500-lb RAF bomb were calculated to riddle with anthrax 10 acres of town or 50 acres in the country. Four thousand 500-lb scatter bombs would do for Stuttgart, 40,350 would finish off the lot, with Aachen and Wilhelmshaven thrown in as a bonus. The 4,000,000 bomblets would be spattered by 2690 bomber-sorties, easily achieved by an air force which a year later could put 1000 planes over Cologne in a night.

Churchill was impressed with the scheme. Anthrax was admittedly not cricket, but neither was war. Any night the church bells of Sussex and Kent might peal the official warning that the Wehrmacht had set jackboots on English shingle. Besides, we needed a tit-for-tat, in case the unspeakable Hitler decided to save himself shot and shell by spraying anthrax all over *us*. The anthrax missile went into production.

This was tricky. A tragic mishap filling the usual sort of bomb meant the end of a factory and perhaps a hundred war workers. With anthrax bomblets, a slip-up was liable in time to decimate the British population.

Then came Pearl Harbor. The might of American ingenuity was unleashed against the dictators (not the Russian one, who had changed sides). While American laboratories poured out penicillin in a flood unimaginable to the British – we were growing it in bedpans and milk churns in the animal house of the pathology school in Oxford – the US Chemical Warfare Service equally efficiently started popping out anthrax bomblets. Berlin, Stuttgart, Frankfurt, Hamburg, Aachen and Wilhelmshaven, they assured their British allies, would be fully taken care of by the Yanks.

Like many of Churchill's clever conceptions – the mighty Hukkabuk floating forts made from ice and wood chips, the oil pipes to set the sea ablaze in 1940 and boil the Germans – the anthrax project saw service no more active than the generals sitting comfortably in Whitehall and the Pentagon. Time is as unkind to man's inventions as to man himself. The glittering technology of one year is the scrap heap of the next. The luxurious *Queen Mary* was ousted by the jet, the chatter of the radio by the glare of TV, tinned peas became frozen, and the backs of envelopes capitulated to the pocket calculator. The murderous inheritance of the anthrax bomb was cruelly usurped by the atom bomb.

Anthrax retained its devotees, like those enthusiasts who puff passionately for steam trains, or race to Brighton in vintage cars. They included Brigadier O. H. Wansbrough-Jones, who wrote to the Chiefs of Staff with charming optimism in 1945, 'Its use in minor wars on which it is not worth using atom bombs, or major ones in which they were being barred, is not impossible.'

Reasons for dropping the atom rather than the anthrax bomb

1. The population of Berlin, Stuttgart, Frankfurt, Hamburg, Aachen and Wilhelmshaven could be reasonably reliably exterminated by six 1945 atom bombs (possibly only five, Frankfurt and Stuttgart being near enough to share). This would need only six Flying Fortress sorties, not 2690 Lancaster sorties.
2. Though the anthrax bomb is considerably quieter, a big bang impresses the enemy tremendously.
3. Anthrax fallout cannot be easily measured with a Geiger counter.

4.   An atom bomb is probably easier to make, is easier to handle and looks better.

5.   Death from an atomic explosion occurs in a milli-second, with anthrax you have to wait a week.

6.   The atom bomb is more warlike. Nobody ever got a medal for spreading disease.

It is fascinating to speculate on the course of world history had Hiroshima been attacked on 6 August 1945 with 1000 tons of anthrax instead.

That summer, man stood amid the rotting bones of his own inhumanity. The horrors exhumed by the allied armies were so widespread and terrible, everyone forgot about the sacrificial sheep of Gruinard. Except Dr Fildes, who had thereby become Sir Paul.

Everyone had also forgotten about the spores. They could lie like murderous Sleeping Beauties in the soil for years. The British Government had forgotten its own Anthrax Order of 1938, decreeing that animals dead from anthrax should be instantly buried on the spot in quicklime, like its executed murderers. At the end of World War Two, on 2 September 1945, the only dangerous place left in Europe was Gruinard Island.

On the mainland, braw men gazed upon it for years and shook timorously over their drams, like kilted Transylvanians round Dracula's castle. Mothers threatened misbehaving bairns with maroonment. The minister preached against it, when he was temporarily short of other evil.

A large back and white metal notice now warns from the shore –

GRUINARD ISLAND

THIS ISLAND IS GOVERNMENT PROPERTY THE
GROUND IS CONTAMINATED AND DANGEROUS
LANDING IS PROHIBITED BY ORDER 1966

This gentle little island, a perch for seabirds, a haven for fish, has like Bikini Atoll been condemned by mankind to solitude for geological life. Worse medical disasters have occurred, but not on Gruinard. It ruined the tourist trade.

On short summer nights when the breeze comes lightly from the northwest, they say you can hear the plaintive, baaing coughing of anthrax-infested sheep.

3

Transatlantic Disaster
The West and Red Indian revenge

24 November 1494 brought the conjunction of Jupiter, Mars and Saturn in the sign of the scorpion. This signalled an imminent outbreak of fearful venereal disease. The soothsayers spoke of little else.

On 21 February 1495, Charles VIII 'The Affable' of France laid siege to Naples. (He did not *really* lay siege, he rode towards Vesuvius amid the tactful cheers of the populace.)

Naples was full of Spanish immigrants. In April 1493, Christopher Columbus had arrived in Barcelona from the Americas. A new disease shortly arrived in Barcelona. It caused spots all over, stinking ulcers, ravaging of the flesh, death, lingering agonies for the survivors. They had to build a special hospital in Seville. Nobody knew what to call it, until Hieronymus Frascastorious of Verona in 1530 hit on 'Syphilis'. This was the young shepherd who picked it up for annoying the gods. Columbus's sailors had picked it up in Haiti.

The Spaniards gave it to the Neopolitans, who called it the Spanish disease, who gave it to the French, who called it the Neapolitan disease and gave it to everybody else. In the scurry to share the blame, the Poles called it the German disease and vice versa, the English (naturally) called it the French disease, and anyone short of foreign suspects could call it the Turkish disease, because the Turks had everything.

Explorers in Columbus's wake discovered the American Indians peacefully puffing their pipes. In 1565, the French ambassador to Lisbon, Jean Nicot, presented an American tobacco plant to Queen Catherine de' Medici, the King's mother, who ran France. He was honoured by her christening it *Nicotina tabacum*.

Soon the pipes were lighting up all over Europe. Tobacco now causes 50,000 deaths a year in Britain, and with Voltairean irony 320,000 a year among the Europeans who sailed to spread themselves across the Redskins' fragrant forests, pure prairies and refreshing rivers. A terrible ransom to extract for violation of privacy.

Thank God America today sends us nothing worse than Coca-Cola.

4

Ironing Out the Bugs in Panama
Colonel Gorgas v. *the US Army*

It was not stout Cortez with a wild surmise about a Panama canal. It was his cousin Alvaro de Saavedra Ceron. It was not even Cortez on 25 September 1513 who star'd silent upon a peak in Darien. It was Balboa, who would have ruined the scansion.

The German Emperor Charles V – he had inherited Spain from his mother – thought a canal the greatest idea since the chastity belt. Frustrated by politics and tormented by gout, Charles abdicated in 1555 to live his last three years in a monastery. His son Philip II declared the canal impious. Those oceans whom God hath set asunder let no man join together. He decreed death even for thinking of it.

Philip was at the time married to Mary Tudor of

England, and like most husbands deeply suspicious of his wife's relatives. The English might perfidiously snatch so extravagant and laboriously dug a trophy – he was probably right, they did it with Suez in 1875.

William Paterson, the Scotsman who founded the Bank of England, in 1698 floated the 'Darien Scheme' from the Bahamas. The Spanish Isthmus would enjoy the infinite benefit of a Scottish colony, becoming a tradesmen's entrance to the Pacific, 'Whereby to Britain would be secured the key to the universe, enabling their possessors to give laws to both oceans and to become arbiters of a commercial world'.

On 26 July the Scots sailed from Leith, christened their wedge of the Isthmus New Caledonia, its unbuilt cities New Edinburgh and New St Andrews. Within a year, starvation, sickness and the Spaniards saw them off. The investors lost all their money, as their many successors with financial schemes conceived in the Bahamas.

Twenty-one-year-old Horatio Nelson first saw active service in 1780, sailing a frigate to San Juan, 250 miles north of Panama in Nicaragua. The expedition was a disaster. Of his 200 crew, 190 died of fever, Nelson himself fell sick and was nearly lost to glory. The trans-Isthmus railway was built in 1855 by Americans William E. Howland and William H. Aspinwall, with the help of Chinese and Irish labourers who died with the near predictability of hogs herded into Chicago slaughterhouses.

In 1876 man and geography were matched.

The Suez Canal had been opened on 17 November 1869 by the Empress Eugénie sailing in the French imperial yacht *Aigle*. Her cousin Ferdinand de Lesseps had become the world's greatest hero since Alexander the Great and its most famous benefactor since the Good Samaritan. If a Frenchman could pierce Suez and Mont Cenis, why should a few sandbanks and lumps of rock frustrate his ravishment of Panama?

In 1876 the Société Civile Internationale du Canal Interocéanique was formed in Paris. In May 1878 it sent

23

Lieutenant L. N. Bonaparte-Wyse to reconnoitre. He brought home the canal concession from the Colombian government. The Société sold it to de Lesseps's Panama Canal Company for ten million francs. On New Year's Day 1880 de Lesseps's little granddaughter administered the first *coup de pioche*, and there was a gala performance at the Panama theatre with Sarah Bernhardt. De Lesseps was seventy-four.

Extravagance, corruption, dishonesty and greed were the canal diggers' unseen enemies. The Colombia courts multiplied land values a thousand times, the French as eagerly paid up. The *Aëdes aegypti* mosquito was their barely visible deadly one. It bore on its wings yellow fever.

The death rate among de Lesseps's men settled down at 176 per thousand. Of 86,800 employees over eight years, 52,814 fell ill and 5627 died. The French found no cold season to kill off the germs. Only the wet season from April to December when you were liable to die in three days from yellow fever, and the dry season from December to April when you were liable to die in twenty-four hours from pernicious fever.

There were 624 deaths in October 1884. Monkey Hill outside Colon became congested with forty funerals a day. A shipment of 500 young French engineers all died in the swamps before they could draw their first month's pay. In September 1884 the entire crew died of yellow fever aboard a British brig anchored off Colon. The French allowed only 0·5 per cent of their budget for hospitals, for sanitation nothing at all. In 1888 the Panama Canal Company went bankrupt.

Nothing is more dangerous than the buckled lance of *amour propre*. Furious France indicted Ferdinand de Lesseps and his son Charles with breach of trust. The Government anyway needed scapegoats to protect the Third Republic from its gleeful enemies. Father and son got five years. Ferdinand was too ill to imprison, he died poor and embittered at La Chenaie on 7 December 1894, a victim of yellow fever, second-hand.

Anthony Froude wrote at the time, 'In all the world there is not perhaps now concentrated in any single spot so much swindling and villainy, so much foul disease, such a hideous dung-heap of physical and moral abomination. The Isthmus is a damp, tropical jungle, intensely hot, swarming with mosquitoes, snakes, alligators, scorpions and centipedes; the home, even as Nature made it, of yellow fever, typhus and dysentery.'

The forty-mile-wide Isthmus was a tangle of vegetation, palms, mangroves and creepers, alive with monkeys, parrots, vividly plumaged birds, wild turkeys, wild boar and hogs, snakes, lizards and tarantulas. Though the flowers were lovely. The orchids had tempted several zealous botanists to their graves. There was frequent lightning, more frequent rain. It was a dank terror abuzz with mosquitoes. Just the challenge for Americans to prove themselves better men than the French.

America needed a Panama Canal to safeguard her national interest as the British needed the Straits of Dover. In February 1904 the Senate ratified a canal treaty with the three-month-old Republic of Panama. It would be dug by the US Corps of Engineers, under an Isthmian Canal Commission headed by Colonel G. W. Goethals. It would cost $156,378,258.

The Americans arrived to find disintegrating French machinery, rusting locomotives growing trees, buildings half-digested by the jungle. Perhaps they felt the neighbourliness with death of Walter Scott's Sergeant More McAlpin, whose habitual morning walk was beneath the elms of the churchyard. New York could proudly call itself 'The Empire State'. Panama had won the title of 'The White Man's Grave'.

In June 1904 Colonel William Crawford Gorgas of the US Army Medical Corps arrived with five other doctors and Miss Hibberd, the nurse. Colonel Gorgas had lived with yellow fever as comfortably as Sherlock Holmes with crime.

Yellow fever is ferocious jaundice. A fulminating,

massive infection of the liver, the body's powerhouse. It starts with rocketing fever, up to 106 degrees Fahrenheit, with backache, headache, photophobia and prostration. Next, bleeding from the mouth, nose and gums, bleeding into the skin, bleeding unseen into the gut. Then the jaundice and vomiting, ending with the notorious 'black vomit' of broken-down blood exuded into the stomach.

The kidneys and the bone marrow go the way of the liver, the patient stops passing urine and making blood cells, turns delirious, slips from convulsions to coma, dies. Yellow fever lurks still in tropical Africa and Central and South America, the traveller safeguarded by immunization with the attenuated living vaccine. The germ is an RNA arbovirus (ribonucleic acid arthropod-borne), its reservoir monkeys. The incubation period is three to six days.

Gorgas was born in 1854 at Mobile, under the stimulating prenatal influence of Dr Josiah Nott, the first to suggest that mosquitoes might possibly spread yellow fever. 'Yellow Jack' was also 'Yellow Breeze', believed to be borne by the wind. Or by oranges and bananas, frenziedly burned by the crateful during epidemics.

Gorgas was medicine's action man. He first wanted to kill people, and tried joining the Army. Throwing his energies into reverse, he graduated from Bellevue Hospital, New York, in 1880. *Then* he joined the Army. His enthusiasm was directed to yellow fever, which had weighed heavily on the military mind since it killed more Americans from 1846 to 1848 than had the Mexicans. Gorgas was posted to Fort Brown, Texas, and placed under arrest for entering the off-limits fever ward.

His colonel's daughter, Miss Doughty Lyster, caught yellow fever. Her own doctor evaluated her chances of recovery by ordering her grave to be dug. Colonel Lyster woefully invited Gorgas – as a professional man, in the lack of a chaplain – to conduct the funeral service. Gorgas brisky agreed, but was forestalled by both the patient getting better and catching yellow fever himself. His attack was slight. He convalesced with Doughty, fell in love and married her, his happiness complete by now being immune to yellow fever for life.

In 1898 Gorgas cleaned up Havana. He believed like everyone else that yellow fever was caused by 'filth', and started vigorously making the place 'as cleanly as Fifth Avenue'. His passion was disastrously misplaced. The yellow fever got worse. Not among the poor Cubans in their insanitary hovels (they were immune). Among the 25,000 settlers from Spain and the United States in their airy spotless dwellings (they were not). Cleanliness seemed as desirable as innocence amid thieves.

The Military Governor died of yellow fever. So did the Chief Commissary of the Army. His widow *wanted* to die of yellow fever, and attempted suttee by rolling in the black vomit which plastered her husband's corpse. It did not work, so she shot herself. The commanding general's staff officer attended her funeral, caught yellow fever and died in four days. It was a dreadful week.

The origin of yellow fever was as baffling as the origin of the universe. You did not catch it from someone, like a cold. How otherwise would the commissary's widow have survived that poisonous vomit? She had no earlier attack and no immunity. (As Queen Victoria had luckily won immunity to typhoid, before she frantically kissed her husband's typhoid-slain corpse at Windsor Castle in 1861.)

There was Dr Henry Carter's mysterious 'period of extrinsic incubation'. You got yellow fever from visiting a friend who was recovering after a fortnight, but never if you compassionately hastened round as soon as he fell sick. There was the ghostly 'Bacillus X', until Surgeon-General Sternberg exorcised it in 1900. Then Dr Carlos Finlay got the idea of mosquitoes.

Dr Finlay was a friend of Gorgas, amiably sceptical of his Operation Fifth Avenue in Havana. Major Walter Reed of Virginia had just arrived there. He thought mosquitoes, too. He had the satisfaction of producing fourteen cases among his friends, by submitting them to mosquito bites or injections of patients' blood. He had seven enlisted men sleep in beds just vacated by yellow fever victims. None got it. His colleague, Dr Jesse W. Lazear, made a sad final sentence to the chapter of yellow fever disasters by dying after an accidental mosquito bite.

The *Aëdes aegypti* mosquito stood indicted and convicted of mass murder. Its criminal *modus operandi* was sucking blood in the first three days of fever, developing the disease in its body and passing it on after twelve. Young mosquitoes which fed by day were seldom infected. The old ones fed at evening and early morning, danger times. A mosquito once infected stayed infective for life. Gorgas threw mosquito-proof screens round his patients and instantly mounted a powerful search-and-destroy operation against mosquitoes. He freed Havana from yellow fever for the first time in 150 years. Then he travelled to the end of the Great American Rainbow in Panama.

Gorgas did not officially exist. He had neither government funds, backing nor encouragement. His sanitary regulations were either rejected or niggardly imposed and ignored by the workers. Admiral J. G. Walker of the Canal Commission knew his own mind. 'I am not going to spend good American dollars on a group of insane enthusiasts who spend their time chasing mosquitoes. Chasing mosquitoes through the Panama jungle seems to me the very height of folly. Even the French in their wildest moments never did anything as bad as that. As everyone knows, what causes yellow fever is not mosquitoes but filth and dirt.'

'Sanitation!' cried General G. W. Davis, first Governor of the Canal Zone. 'What has that to do with digging the canal? Spending a dollar on sanitation is as good as throwing it into the Bay. It's for your own good, Gorgas, I say this,' he advised benevolently. 'You have harped on the mosquito idea until it has become an obsession, and your assistants have caught it, too. Oh do, for goodness sake get it out of your head! Yellow fever, as we all know, is caused by filth.'

Colonel Goethals himself was more analytical. 'Do you

28

know, Gorgas, that every mosquito you kill costs the US Government ten dollars?'

'But just think, Colonel Goethals,' Gorgas replied pleasantly. 'One of those ten-dollar mosquitoes might bite you, and what a loss that would be to the country.'

A hideous, swiftly fatal disease borne by gossamer-winged mosquitoes! As ridiculous to men who thought of death in terms of batteries and battleships as the suggestion of man-eating butterflies. The French failed at Panama through mismanagement and waste. The Americans would win through stringent economy. These robust sentiments were all uttered in Washington, DC. The Commission saw no reason for visiting Panama. They might catch yellow fever.

There was no yellow fever when Gorgas arrived at Panama in June 1904. The disease had left with the French. There were no susceptible strangers to catch it. December saw 6 cases and 1 death. January 1905, 19 cases and 8 deaths. On New Year's Eve, officers of the US cruiser *Boston* in Colon harbour had thrown a party. One mild case of yellow fever was unknowingly invited, a fortnight later six of the crew went down. April brought 9 cases and 2 deaths. May, 33 cases, 8 deaths. In June there were 62 cases and 19 deaths. In July there was panic.

An epidemic! Everyone wanted to go home. Engineers, clerks, cooks, labourers, shopkeepers. The canal could be abandoned. The greatest American dream since Independence itself was vanishing through the everyday disaster of not doing what your doctor told you.

But they could not go home. The only escape from Panama was by water, as from Alcatraz. There were no ships. By the time a rescue flotilla was mustered they might all be dead. They could only stare at each other with a wild surmise they might be developing yellow fever. They began to consider that there might be something in those goddam mosquitoes after all.

Gorgas swung into action.

If you wanted water in Panama, you had to wait until

29

it rained. It was collected and stored near the houses in an infinite variety of domestic utensils. The mosquitoes laid eggs on the water – the outbreak aboard the *Boston* came from a purée of mosquito larvae in a pan outside the galley. Gorgas's restive memory recalled that yellow fever vanished from New York when the water vanished into pipes. Eliminate standing water, eliminate yellow fever.

Colonel Gorgas divided his forces. The *Aëdes* Brigade would attack the mosquitoes of yellow fever. The *Anopheles* Brigade those of malaria. He established the criminal offence of harbouring mosquito larvae, fine five dollars. A mosquito needs little room for reproduction. Crevices in stones, thrown-out cans, holy water stoups in churches, all made love nests. An outbreak in the hospital was traced to the little dishes of water at the legs of the food safe, to keep out the ants.

Gorgas advanced on the vegetation with flame throwers. The captured enemy was chloroformed and microscoped, to determine its precise regiment in the swarming army. All patients were camouflaged with mosquito netting. A phone call to the sanitary squad, reporting marauding mosquitoes, instantly produced a truck with a sanitary inspector and half a dozen men, crawling all over your house with flashlights. You would not get that sort of service today, even reporting a cellarful of dead rats.

In a brilliant strategic stroke, Gorgas deployed large, flat, scoured pans of fresh water, so inviting that the *Aëdes aegypti* mosquitoes hastened to lay their eggs – then Gorgas outwitted the foe by tipping the lot down the disinfected drain. The yellow fever mosquito fancied clean water and bred close to houses. The malaria mosquito bred anywhere. Gorgas vigorously drained the swamps. There was hardly a puddle left. Panama had eight million feet of ditches, and every stream painstakingly polluted with a film of oil.

In September 1906, Gorgas – no firefly under a bushel – boasted, 'In six months I have rid the Isthmus of yellow fever – after four hundred years!' Then Secretary of War Taft fired him.

During 1906, the American Medical Association sent Dr Charles Reed snooping round Panama. The AMA entertained doubts about the collaboration of the Isthmian Commission with its medical staff.

Dr Reed discovered that if – say – the superintendent of Ancon Hospital in Panama needed supplies, he sent the appropriate form to the chief sanitary officer, who sent it to the Governor of the Zone, who sent it to the chief disbursing officer, who sent it to the Isthmian Canal Commission, who sent it to a member of the Commission detailed to specialize in such things, who sent it back to the Isthmian Canal Commission, who, if they approved of it, invited bids from contractors by sending it to their purchasing agent, who was not expected to know anything about sanitation, who sent the article to the Isthmus c/o the chief of the Bureau of Materials and Supplies, who – the pace now hots up – sent it to the chief disbursing officer who had first mailed the form to the Commission, who passed the consignment to Colonel Gorgas, who presented it to the hospital superintendent, if he was lucky. Up-and-coming America in Panama was determined to muddle through as steadfastly as complacent Britain in the Crimea. Gorgas and the vigorous Miss Nightingale would have made a lovely couple.

Teddy Roosevelt got to hear, and changed the system. He also made all Commission members go and live in Panama. The President had earlier appointed Governor Shonts there. Shonts wanted to replace Gorgas with a friend of his own in the medical line, an osteopath. Quite right, agreed Mr Secretary Taft, who concurred with Governor Shonts that the cause of yellow fever was bad smells. Taft had sniffed for himself, and Panama smelt as bad as ever. All Gorgas did in Panama was to endanger the success of the entire scheme.

This could have been the most disastrous disaster of all. Gorgas went, but luckily his work remained. The death rate in the Canal Zone by 1914 was 6·2 per thousand, compared with that of the entire United States 14·1 per thousand.

William Gorgas died on 3 July 1920 at Queen Alexandra's Military Hospital, Millbank, London. He was visiting the capital of so much potentially pestiferous land that the sun never set on it.

King George V had made him a knight (honorary). The British gave him St Paul's for his funeral. His country buried him in Arlington. Gorgas has been meanly criticized as a scientist who never discovered, but won his reputation from the discoveries of others. He fulfilled completely the remark of his contemporary physician, Sir William Osler of Oxford – 'In science the credit goes to the man who convinces the world, not the man to whom the idea first occurs.'

On Thursday, 20 November 1913 the first ship sailed through the canal. She was the French *Louise* which twenty-five years before had taken de Lesseps back to France. Brash America was determined to make a *beau geste* as handsomely as polished France.

The finished canal followed the same route as suggested by Alvaro de Saavedra Ceron in 1523.

5

Surgical Souvenirs
Litigious litter

These operative oversights were reported to a doctors' legal insurance society in London over eighteen years.

	Swabs left inside	All articles (instruments, needles, etc.) left inside
1962	38	41
1963	27	45
1964	37	68
1965	32	54
1966	31	52
1967	30	41
1968	26	39
1969	25	46
1970	21	28
1971	33	56
1972	31	60
1973	25	30
1974	20	35
1975	25	46
1976	26	45
1977	21	90
1978	18	60
1979	16	110
Totals	482	946

Surgeons are becoming no less forgetful.

More gruesomely, a large forceps used for holding swabs – acting like scissors with locking handles, measuring 9½ inches by 3 – was discovered in the ashes of a woman aged 76 a week after operation on her kidney. The operation wound itself was only 7 inches long and 3½ inches deep. It could never have concealed the forceps. No instruments were missing in the operating theatres or the sterile supply store. No one ever knew how it accompanied her to the furnace.

6

The Green Monkeys
Revenge in the Rhineland

In August 1967, a cargo of African green monkeys was flown from Entebbe in Uganda to Frankfurt in West Germany. They made a stopover in the African–South American room of the Royal Society for the Prevention of Cruelty to Animals' hostel at Heathrow Airport, London.

The green-, yellow- or black-furred vervet monkey *Cercopithecus aethiops* was a regular airline passenger. A quarter of a million of them had entered Europe and the United States to participate in laboratory research. Their kidneys were wonderful for growing viruses in test tubes.

The consignment was booked to Marburg, a university town fifty miles north of Frankfurt, where Luther and Zwingli in 1529 disputed on transubstantiation. Shortly after the monkeys' arrival, staff at the Behringverke Pharmaceutical Company, and at the Paul-Ehrlich Institute in Frankfurt, were struck by an illness unknown to man.

They developed sudden fever, headache, vomiting, watery diarrhoea, widespread pains. They became covered with tiny bright red spots, with reddening of the scrotum or vulva, and blisters in mouth and throat. The liver enlarged, the sex glands were inflamed, the kidney faltered, the heart softened, the brain swelled. Blood oozed from nose, gums, gut, bladder, even the pricks of syringes. A second batch of patients appeared among the doctors, nurses and families of the first. Thirty-one people caught it, seven died.

It was an alarming disease, even for the uninfected. Nobody at first knew the cause, the treatment, the chances of recovery, how catching it was, how dangerous. Would it ravage susceptible, overpopulated Europe, making the Black Death look like a minor accident?

The original patients had handled the green monkeys, either living, dead or sliced. What made these monkeys unlike their quarter of a million harmless little fellows? The answer came from the British germ warfare centre at Porton Down, still busy. Materially, this is isolated in the most beautiful country of southern England. Psychologically, it shares a menacing landscape with atomic power stations and atomic waste dumps, particularly if viewed from the left.

Porton Down calmed the panic by isolating an unknown virus, unusually long with a hook on the end, resembling a spanner. They could grow it on cells from baby hamster kidneys or from the human foreskin.

The Marburg monkeys were meanwhile traced to the Lake Kyoga region, north of Kampala, all from the same monkey trapper. The disease they carried to Europe was not even a symptomless monkey disease. Doctors proved this by injecting green monkeys with the virus and finding the lot died.

All admittedly hard luck on the monkeys. The sensitive and high-minded, who revolt against such experiments on animals for the benefit of us all, should know their two most powerful allies this century – it was in evidence at a Nuremberg trial – were Adolf Hitler and Hermann Goering.

The Marburg virus probably lives naturally in a rare central African animal or plant, being transferred to the monkeys by the bite of some insect – the funnel-webbed spider was suspect. The outbreak was quelled, but the disease could recur virulently anywhere in the world.

The lives the green monkeys took from man saved an infinite number of their own. They are now highly unpopular in civilization's laboratories.

35

7

A Touch of Class
Waiting-room disaster

In 1661, Charles II granted a charter to the Royal Society for Improving Natural Knowledge (a founder member was Sir Christopher Wren). He contributed valuably to medical science by increasing the annual ration of hanged criminals for dissection by the Royal College of Surgeons from four to six. He was simultaneously the biggest buff among English monarchs for the Royal Touch to cure the King's Evil (scrofula – swollen tuberculous glands of the neck). This worked as the touch of God, percolated through the divine right of kings. It was performed ceremoniously with choirs, Beefeaters, and ladies- and gentlemen-in-waiting. Charles treated 92,107 patients. The rush was once so great that six were trampled to death.

8

Boob Boobs
A thing of beauty is a joy for lawyers

If you do not care for just the way you look tonight, a plastic surgeon can operate on you as efficiently as a fairy godmother on toads.

Take your choice of cut.

Facelift
Camouflage incision under hairline, pull taut, insert tuck, snip off selvedge. Eliminates the sags like wind in your sails.

Nosebob

All done from inside. Makes a classical feature of something fit only as a perch for glasses.

Browbob

Eliminates furrows by cut at nape of neck, scalp pulled back, surplus sliced, secured with metal staples as for sealing postal packets. Stops you looking worried.

Boobbob

Any shape from Rubens to Bernard Buffet, Picasso if you like.

Wattlebob

Turns old turkeys into fighting cocks.

Bagbob

Under eyes, cancels a lifetime's dissipation.

Bumbob

Goes with Tummy Tuck, Thigh Whittling, Fat Syphoning. Anything is preferable to dieting.

Hair Transplant

Replaces bald patches with flourishing ones, as returfing the lawn.

Plastic surgery like any other has its mistakes, but they are more obvious. The facelift droops with time, as an uneaten soufflé. Surgeons favour a standard, quick, pert nose job, and a woman is more infuriated encountering another wearing the same little nose as the same little dress. Boob-boosting is done with silicone implants, which can slop like sandbags to cause severe list to port or starboard. This once brought thunderous applause, occurring suddenly at the climax of a stripper's act.

Mrs Virginia O'Hare of New York said she wanted a

flat, sexy belly. The plastic surgeon left her navel 1½ inches off centre. She sued him, won the disastrous damages of $650,000. This operative error is priced at $433,333 per inch, or over fifteen and a half million dollars a yard.

9

Rude Awakening

Frozen assets

A clammy summer night in the accident department. Young man in T-shirt and jeans lies screened on a couch. He was brought in by ambulance deeply unconscious.

The houseman is new, young, female, pretty, clever. She doubts the diagnosis. He responds perfectly normally to the appropriate tests. *Is he shamming?* Is he really wide awake? People *do* behave so oddly in hospitals.

Doctor and nurse confer. 'Why not,' suggests the nurse sensibly, 'spray his genitals with ethyl chloride? *That* will show pretty smartly if he's swinging the lead.'

Excellent idea!

Ethyl chloride is a colourless liquid, highly volatile, once popular as a rough-and-ready local anaesthetic. Instant evaporation when sprayed on the skin produces a frozen numbness, enough for operations like opening abcesses, removing small warts, piercing ears.

Doctor and nurse unzip their patient's flies, retract his Y-fronts, take aim, spray. The action is spectacular. A fine, frosty film forms on the skin, like the bloom on deep-frozen meatballs.

Instant effect.

Patient jumps up, pulls together clothes, storms from hospital.

Case not concluded. A hot letter complains of his privates getting a cold shower. Disastrous litigation avoided by hospital diplomatically insisting that he had after all suffered no harm in the two ladies' hands.

He agreed.

A lot of men might quite like it.

10

Typhoid Mary
Death on a plate

'The cook was a good cook, as cooks go; and as cooks go she went,' Saki wrote in 1904. Mary Mallon was then traversing the spacious, moneyed houses of New York State. She had eight jobs in seven years. Among seven families, her tenure coincided with a nasty outbreak of typhoid fever.

At Marnaroneck in 1900, a young man who came to stay in September got typhoid ten days later. Mary spent 1901 in New York City. The household laundress died of typhoid in Roosevelt Hospital just before Christmas. Next summer took her to Dark Harbor, Maine, into a lawyer's household of eight, seven down with typhoid in a fortnight. The lawyer was immune from an earlier attack. Mary devoted herself to the sick so unsparingly he gave her an extra $50.

She moved in 1904 to Sands Point, Long Island. Typhoid broke out a week later, four cases out of ten, all domestics. The New York City Health Department decided there was something mysteriously noxious about the servants' quarters. Typhoid exploded a week after Mary's arrival at Oyster Bay on Long Island Sound in 1909 (six out of ten, three family, three servants). While Colonel Gorgas was boasting he had freed Panama from yellow fever, New York City suffered that year 3467 cases of typhoid with 639 deaths.

The disease seldom seeped from the city into Oyster Bay. Dr George A. Soper hurried from New York, busied himself with the milk, the water, the family fare, the well and the cesspool, the cistern and the privy, the manure spread on the lawn. What did they like most to eat? Clams. Clams! Typhoid grenades. For sure, it was the fault of that old Indian woman who lived on the beach and peddled clams at the back door.

Typhoid is patchy inflammation of the small intestine, which coils in the abdomen like an inflated condom six feet long. The patient develops steadily rising fever, a fleeting rash, bellyache, cough, greenish diarrhoea (the 'staircase temperature, rose spots and pea-soup stools' of florid Edwardian physicians). Today it is cured with the antibiotic chloramphenicol. In the time of Typhoid Mary, as with most illnesses, you either got better or died according to your luck.

The germs have long hairlike flagellae, and can scuttle about. A tiny dose can bring a widespread epidemic, through water, food, milk, flies. These are contaminated by the faeces of a carrier who has recovered from the disease, perhaps an attack too mild to identify. In the 1900s, this conception of apparently healthy carriers first explained the mysterious scattering of typhoid epidemics. One typhoid patient in twenty continues excreting live bacteria for a year. Some, intermittently for life. These are nearly all women.

Luckily for the Indian's trade, nobody in the Oyster Bay house had eaten clams for six weeks, well outside the incubation period. What else did they enjoy? asked Dr Soper. The cook's ice cream was delicious. Oh, not the present cook. The one who left suddenly, three weeks after the typhoid started.

Dr Soper found the cook six months later. He traced her through Tuxedo NY (one case) to Park Avenue (two servants suffering typhoid, the daughter of the house dead with it).

Mary Mallon was forty, unmarried, an immigrant from Northern Ireland. She had thick greying hair, round steel-rimmed glasses, straight full eyebrows, a placid face with a mouth turned down at the corners. Her fat figure was a good reference. She was shy, surly, sullen and secretive.

They met in the kitchen. Dr Soper tactfully suggested some connection between these sickly visitations and her floury fingers. She attacked him with a cleaver. He bolted, and hastened to the New York Health Commissioner, who called the police. Mary gave them the slip. They were leaving when a policeman spotted a scrap of striped skirt caught in a neighbouring privy door. They piled ashcans against it, and called her to surrender. She came out fighting. Biting, screaming, kicking, she was removed in a motor ambulance, an inspector from the City Health Department sitting on her chest.

They took Mary to the Riverside Hospital for communicable diseases on North Brother Island, 13 acres in the East River off the Bronx, facing Rikers Island with its gaol. The press fed on her with relish. Mary was drawn as a comic-strip witch, dropping skulls into the pot, sizzling on the stove typhoid bacilli the size of frankfurters. The public was hysterical. How many malevolent Marys were there, murdering New Yorkers without the inconvenience of breaking the law?

Dr Soper took a swab from her stools, incubated it, and looked down his microscope. Teeming with typhoid bacilli. He explained patiently she had a fatal disease, for other people. Typhoid germs were breeding in her gall-bladder as cosily as bees in a hive. The cure was straightforward – removal of gall-bladder.

Mary had no spark of the dazzling altruism which blinded the fabled Pole afflicted with the evil eye, who put out his sight lest he harm his children. She refused. Quite rightly, too. A cholecystectomy in 1907 was as uninviting as a heart transplant today. Dr Soper suggested the less painful alternative of abandoning cooking. She objected that cooking was her livelihood, a skill affording her pride and delight. They kept her in Riverside for three years.

Mary was a morose prisoner-patient, angry, rebellious, threatening, certain she was a victim of a doctors' plot. She

41

refused to admit, perhaps even to believe, that she was a typhoid carrier. She worked as a hospital laundress, winning her release in 1910 with a promise to stay at the copper instead of the cooker, and to report three-monthly to the Health Department.

She disappeared. She became Mrs Brown, the cook. She was not like a gaolbird heartlessly resuming dangerous crime as a familiar living. She was expressing her independence, her defiance, her resentment towards fellow humans who fearfully accused her of casting spells.

For five years Mary worked unsuspected in the kitchens of New York. Typhoid cases followed her as surely as crows carrion. The disease was too commonplace for anxious speculation on each source. In 1915 a serious epidemic affected the staff of the Sloane Hospital for Women, New York (25 cases, 2 deaths). The kitchenmaids called the cook 'Typhoid Mary' for a joke. She fled. When the police found her working on Long Island, she went quietly.

Mary returned to North Brother Island. She had earned herself the sentence of quarantine for life. The Health Department could never risk freeing again the newspapers' ghoul of the griddle. Even embittered typhoid carriers mellow with age. Gradually Mary accepted possessing the guiltless danger of a hungry tiger at large. She went over to the enemy, working as a Riverside laboratory technician. New York, too, became kindlier. In 1923 the city built her a cottage beside the hospital, where she gave tea parties.

Mary had a stroke on Christmas Day 1932. She never walked again. Riverside cared for her tenderly. She got religion. She never spoke of family or birthplace. Typhoid was an unmentionable subject. She died on 11 November 1938 of bronchopneumonia complicating chronic nephritis and myocarditis, excreting typhoid to the last.

Her official score was 53 cases and 3 deaths. Her unattributed ones were vastly more. Hers was probably the 1903 epidemic of 1400 cases at Ithaca in upstate New York.

Mary Mallon was America's first named typhoid carrier. When she died, 300 were known in New York, all prevented from working with food or water. The title of 'New York Carrier No. 1' escaped her. When there were sufficient to warrant a list, Mary came alphabetically No. 36.

Only nine people went to her funeral. Every doctor in the world knows her name.

11

Disastrous Motherhood

Tales from the Vienna wards

The Autocrat of the Breakfast Table was superbly dictatorial on 13 February 1843.

> A physician holding himself in readiness to attend cases of midwifery should never take any active part in the post-mortem examination of cases of puerperal fever.
>
> If a physician is present at such autopsies, he should use thorough ablution, change every article of dress, and allow twenty-four hours or more to elapse before attending to any case of midwifery. It may be well to extend the same caution to cases of simple peritonitis.
>
> On the occurrence of a single case of puerperal fever in his practice, the physician is bound to consider the next female he attends in labour, unless some weeks at least have elapsed, as in danger of being infected by him. . . . The time has come when the existence of a private pestilence in the sphere of a single physician should be looked upon not as a misfortune but a crime.

Dr Oliver Wendell Holmes was addressing the Boston Society for Medical Improvement. His suggested simple improvement of washing the hands in chloride of lime before delivering the child outraged obstetricians, particularly in Philadelphia.

43

Countered the autocrat, 'Medical logic does not appear to be taught or practised in our schools.'

Surgeons operated in blood-stiffened frock coats – the stiffer the coat, the prouder the busy surgeon – hanging on pegs at the theatre door with *boutonnières* of waxed hemp stitches. Pus was as inseparable from surgery as blood. The yellow ooze from every wound was cheerfully classified as 'laudable pus', 'sanious pus' was unwelcome and 'ichorous pus' the stinking herald of cadaverous putrefaction.

Cleanliness was next to prudishness. 'There was no object in being clean,' later wrote Sir Frederick 'Elephant Man' Treves. 'Indeed, cleanliness was out of place. It was considered to be finicking and affected. An executioner might as well manicure his nails before chopping off a head.'

Puerperal fever terrorized the week after labour. The mother suddenly felt ill, shook with rigors. The lochia discharging from her vagina turned stinking and bloody. Peritonitis developed, thrombosis in the legs, abcesses in the breasts, infection of the lungs and brain, bleeding into the skin, stupor and death. Hippocrates had marked it a disease generally fatal and mysteriously transmitted.

In 1846, Ignaz Philipp Semmelweis was appointed assistant in the First Obstetric Clinic at the Allgemeine Krankenhaus, Vienna. He was short, bald, elegantly moustached, sensitive, excitable, aged twenty-eight, Hungarian. The vast general hospital was built by Empress Maria Theresa, among her bounties to her motley people after the Peace of Paris ended the Seven Years War in 1763.

It encompassed the biggest lying-in hospital in the world. This was divided into the First Clinic, five wards for teaching medical students, and the adjoining Second Clinic, another five for teaching midwives. The mortality from puerperal fever in the First was three times that in the Second.

This was all round Vienna. Weeping women implored their confinement in the Second Clinic. The gloom of childbirth in the First was deepened by its remoteness from the hospital chapel – the last sacrament was borne directly to the dying in the Second Clinic, but to reach the sick room of the First robed priests needed to troop through all five wards behind their tolling bell. Elsewhere in the hospital once a day sufficed, but twenty-four hours is a long time in puerperal fever, and the doomful parade became as familiar among the fearful women as the street sausage vendors.

Semmelweis could pick only one path down the mortality gradient. It led the First Clinic's students to perform vaginal examinations direct from the dissecting room, casually washing their fingers in between. The midwives of the Second Clinic took a cleaner journey to work.

On 20 March 1847, Semmelweis's colleague, Jacobus Kolletschka, Professor of Medical Jurisprudence, died after his finger was wounded by a student while together they cut up a corpse. The professor's riven body in the post-mortem room inspired Semmelweis that the disease which killed professor and countless new mothers was the same.

'Day and night the vision of Kolletschka's malady haunted me', Semmelweis wrote. 'It was not the wound, but the wound rendered unclean by cadaveric material, which had produced the fatal result . . . I must therefore put this question to myself; did then the individuals whom I have seen die from an identical disease also have cadaveric matter carried into the vascular system? To this question I must answer, Yes!'

Every mother had a wound. It was the raw womb which had shed its placenta in the afterbirth.

He ordered his students to wash their hands in chloride of lime. The mortality in the First Clinic fell from 18 per cent to 1 per cent. Semmelweis bettered Oliver Wendell Holmes in perceiving puerperal fever as a poisoning of the blood. He discovered that European doctors could better American ones in bigotry. Semmelweis retired to Budapest.

On 31 July 1865, Semmelweis's friend Ferdinant Hebra

found some pretext of enticing him from his wife and infant to the local madhouse. The intention was to keep him there – sadly, but necessarily, as a patient. The asylum doctor noticed a small wound on a right finger, incurred at Semmelweis's last operation. It turned gangrenous, ate into the finger joint, infection spread up the arm, abcesses formed in the lungs, Semmelweis died on 13 August from the equivalent of puerperal fever.

The disease is no longer in the index of obstetrical textbooks.

12

Disastrous Habits
Tom Brown's schooldays

Thomas Hughes's glorification of public-school life appeared simultaneously in 1857 with Dr William Acton's damnation of its popular DIY activity.

> The frame is stunted and weak, the muscles underdeveloped, the eye is sunken and heavy, the complexion is sallow, pasty, or covered with spots of acne, the hands are damp and cold, and the skin moist. The boy shuns the society of others, creeps about alone, joins with repugnance in the amusements of his schoolfellows. He cannot look anyone in the face, and becomes careless in dress and uncleanly in person. His intellect has become sluggish and enfeebled, and if his evil habits are persisted in, he may end in becoming a drivelling idiot or a peevish valetudinarian. Such boys are to be seen in all stages of degeneration, but what we have described is but the result towards which they all are tending. . . .
>   The pale complexion, the emaciated form, the slouching gait, the clammy palm, the glassy or leaden

eye, and the averted gaze, indicate the lunatic victim
to this vice. Apathy, loss of memory, abeyancy of
concentrative power and manifestation of mind
generally, combined with loss of self-reliance, and
indisposition for or impulsiveness of action, irritability
of temper, and incoherence of language, are the most
characteristic mental phenomena of chronic dementia
resulting from masturbation. . . .

The man will and must pay the penalty for the
errors of the boy; that for one that escapes, ten will
suffer; that an awful risk attends abnormal substitutes
for sexual intercourse; and that self-indulgence, long
pursued, tends ultimately, if carried far enough, to
early death or self-destruction.

Thus *The Function and Disorders of the Reproductive Organs,
in Childhood, Youth, Adult Age, and Advanced Life, Considered in
their Physiological, Social and Moral Relations.* Dr Acton wrote
as well, *Prostitution, Considered in its Moral, Social, and Sanitary
Aspects, in London and other Large Cities and Garrison Towns,
with Proposals for the Control and Prevention of its Attendant
Evils.* Also, *Unmarried Wet-Nurses.*

I doubt if he would have appreciated Dorothy Parker's
scriptural joke, when she named her untidy canary Onan.

13

Scurvy Treatment

Disastrous diet for gallant gentlemen

'The Great War, for instance, could never have happened
if tinned food had not been invented,' said George Orwell.
All his insights were, of course, equally shrewd, but some
more equally than others.

Without tinned food, adventurous polar exploration certainly could never have happened.

47

On 19 May 1845, Captain Sir John Franklin, veteran of Copenhagen and Trafalgar at nineteen, sailed from Greenhithe in the Thames with HMS *Erebus* and *Terror* on his third Arctic expedition. The Admiralty had dispatched him to find the Northwest Passage. There would be a reward of £20,000.

Franklin provisioned for 137 men over 1092 days. Each ship had a library of 1200 books, volumes of *Punch*, and a barrel organ which played fifty different tunes, including ten hymns. His lavish stores included 33,289 pounds of preserved meat, Goldner Patent brand in red tins.

Canning is as old as America. Frenchman Nicholas Appert in the eighteenth century preserved food by heat in sealed jars. Donkin and Hall of Blue Anchor Road in London's dockland were soon supplying the world with tinned mutton and peas, boiled beef and carrots. (The roast veal of 1818 was enjoyed 120 years later by a venturesome English professor.) The Admiralty ordered tinned meat aboard their ships as 'medical comforts'. Fresh-cooked meat would surely cure the scurvy.

Scurvy was a mysterious and terrible peril of the sea. The swollen, bloody, stinking gums, bruised skin, aching bones, sudden death, were thought a contagion among men crammed into ships, camps, besieged cities. In the convict hulks off Woolwich scurvy matched the hangman in efficiency. Or the cause was sea air, fit only for fish. Or it was punishment for laziness, lassitude being an early symptom.

The cure was found in 1597, scurvy-grass. God was well known to have given man diseases and a herb to cure each. The concept of scurvy from *lack* of scurvy-grass was persistently beyond medical imagination, even into this century.

Sir Richard (South Seas) Hawkins cured scurvy in 1793 with oranges and lemons. Seven years later, the East India Company issued all its ships with lemon juice. In 1773, naval surgeon James Lind of Edinburgh published *A Treatise of the Scurvy*, comparable in perception to William Harvey's treatise on the heart.

A year after Lind's death in 1794, and two hundred after Sir Richard Hawkins's idea, the Admiralty responded to Lind's urgings and provided lemon juice. The cases of scurvy in Haslar Naval Hospital dropped in ten years from 1750 to one. Like Lister with hospital gangrene, Lind effected the cure without needing to know the cause.

Sir John Franklin sailed with 9300 pounds of lemon juice in kegs, protected from freezing with a dash of rum. Each man took an ounce a day, sweetened and diluted, swallowed in the presence of an officer.

When he had been away six and a half years, people began to worry. After eight, further search was abandoned for an expedition provisioned only for three. On 20 January 1854, its officers and men were deemed to have died in Her Majesty's service.

Why, no one knew.

That October, Dr John Rae of the Hudson Bay Company heard from Eskimos of thirty-five dead white men near the mouth of Great Fish River in King William Land, a hundred-mile-long island well west of Baffin Land. Franklin's expedition had reached the eastern limits of the expeditions from the Pacific. He had succeeded. He had discovered that the Northwest Passage existed.

Dr Rae hastened to London with spoons, forks, relics of the men. The war had sucked British shipping to the Crimea. It was left for the Hudson Bay Company to organize a search party, which found seven hundred empty meat tins, arranged in regular rows. It seemed that Sir John Franklin had discovered his meat rotten, frantically ordered tin after tin broached, seen his expedition doomed by starvation. Britain erupted, particularly as the stuff was tinned in Galatz, Moravia.

Lady Franklin bought a steam yacht and mounted her own expedition. It discovered that *Erebus* and *Terror* had been trapped in the ice and abandoned on 22 April 1848, 105 survivors reaching shore. Sir John had died on 11 June 1847, aged sixty-one. Scurvy did for the rest.

The cooked meats and vegetables, though fresh in their

tins, had no antiscorbutic vitamin C. This is destroyed by
heat. The decomposing lemon juice was left aboard. The
ships were plundered by the Eskimos and never seen again.

The Eskimos told of white men bleeding from the mouth,
too weak to pull their sledges, struggling for the mainland
of Canada. Vitamin C is synthesized by all animals except
guineapigs and primates. Had the survivors caught fish
and shot the Arctic deer and musk cattle – not for nour-
ishment but for their vitamins – they could have survived.
US army Lieutenant Frederick Schwatka found their bones
in 1878.

Sir John Franklin knew nothing about vitamins. Sir
Frederick Gowland Hopkins of Cambridge won the Nobel
Prize in 1929 for inventing them. In 1932, vitamin C was
found chemically to be ascorbic acid. People now swallow
it by the handful in the touching belief it keeps away colds.

14

The Emperor's Sore Throat

Sir Morell Mackenzie and the Kaiser

At Queen Victoria's Jubilee in 1887, the world looked as
beautiful for Germany as fifty-three years later. Denmark
had been crushed, Austria pulverized and France flattened.

Reichskanzler Bismarck ran an unflinchingly efficient
empire bossed by Prussia. The Crown Princess was Victoria's eldest child, Viki. Her thirty-year-old son William
– his left arm was paralysed from an undiagnosed birth
injury – was Victoria's favourite grandchild. To the Queen
of England, foreign affairs were family affairs, conducted
with letters full of state secrets to eight of her nine children
married into European courts. Her foreign secretaries could
only quake with the impotent horror of the House of Peers
towards the Fairy Queen in *Iolanthe*.

The German Emperor William I had turned ninety.

Viki's husband Frederick, compassionate, democratic, earnest, war-hating, intended to thwart Bismarck and rule the thirty-nine German states linked in peaceful, liberal brotherhood. Princess Viki thought anyone mad who was blind to the overpowering advantages of the British Constitution. She was *die Engländerin*, distrusted and hated. William of the upswept moustaches was Prussian from the spike of his helmet to the click of his heels, and fitted comfortably into Bismarck's tunic pocket.

Among these worms at the kernel of Europe was dropped a pigheaded, humourless, self-satisfied, pushy, middle-aged Scot, who beheld the world through a shilling-sized throat mirror.

That January, stolid, bearded, fifty-five-year-old Crown Prince Frederick grew hoarse. It was ascribed to a nasty cold caught when his coachman became lost in the dark among the mountains, and the Prince had no overcoat. The aromatic inhalations, the tangy gargles, were useless. His physician Dr Wegner, Deputy Medical Director of the Germany Army, called in Professor Gerhardt, the throat man from Berlin.

The professor sprayed cocaine and observed through his mirror a pink nodule on the left vocal chord. He tried pulling it off with a wire snare. No good. He thrust down a knife. No good, either. He sent for the electric cautery and sizzled. The lump got bigger. The professor attacked with the cautery every day for a fortnight. Frederick's motto was *Lerne zu leiden ohne zu klagen* – we must learn to suffer without complaint.

The wound refused to heal. The professor thought vaguely of cancer. But the vocal chords moved normally, which every doctor at the time knew excluded malignancy. Every doctor at the time was disastrously wrong. He prescribed a fortnight at a spa.

The hoarseness grew worse. Gerhardt decided to split open the Adam's apple and look. He called in Professor von Bergmann to do the cutting, physicians then utilizing surgeons as householders plumbers. The operation was fixed among the doctors for 7 a.m. on Saturday, 21 May. With the stealth of scaffold and executioners, operating table and nurses were brought from the Charité Hospital in Berlin to the Neue Palais at Potsdam, which had no bathrooms.

Bismarck discovered with fury they were about to chloroform the Heir Apparent without telling himself, the old Emperor or even the patient. He instantly dispatched reinforcements, Dr Schrader, Professor Tobold, Dr Hahn and Dr von Lauer, who could pull rank as Dr Wegner's commander in the Army. Uneasy lies the head that wears a crown, on a pillow with a circus of doctors round it.

Late that night, Queen Victoria's doctor James Reid, an Aberdonian who resembled a bewhiskered hard-boiled egg, appeared unexpectedly in Dr Morell Mackenzie's bric-à-brac stuffed consulting room at No. 19, Harley Street, London.

The Queen had passed a frightful day. Two frantic telegrams, a distracted letter from Viki, revealed the alarming intention of removing from outside the neck a suspicious, perhaps cancerous, growth in the throat of *unser Fritz*. Viki implored instant dispatch of the celebrated Dr Mackenzie. 'We cannot bear to think of poor darling Viki's anguish and sorrow,' cried the Queen. (She was far more emotional, more vivacious than the statue of her memory. Her evergreen rod, 'We are not amused', swished an equerry telling a spicy story over dinner at Windsor – but maybe he had been loyally following Her Majesty's habit of lacing her claret with Scotch.)

The German doctors had already startled Mackenzie that afternoon with a telegram to join the team. Perhaps they wanted to dilute responsibility. Perhaps they recognized he knew more about the throat then they did. To travel in the purple of the Queen's authority he found electrifying.

Mackenzie was sharp-nosed, thin-lipped, hollow-cheeked, neatly sidewhiskered, in wing collar and frock coat. He smelt of stramonium, taken in cigarettes for his asthma. His practice was so busy, urgent patients needed to tip his butler for priority. In 1887, you lost your tonsils sitting conscious in a high-backed chair, the operator wandering off to puff a throat with powder, to prescribe a gargle or two, before reappearing to mop up the blood.

Mackenzie's dinner table attracted Henry Irving, Beerbohm Tree, Ellen Terry, Pinero and James McNeill Whistler (Whistler's mother's other son was a London throat doctor). His profession despised him as an adventurer. The Royal College of Surgeons regarded his Throat Hospital – still flourishing at Golden Square in Soho – as the Bank of England regarded a pawnbroker's.

Arrived at Potsdam, Mackenzie plunged his own forceps down the patient's throat. The fragments went to Professor Virchow, the world-famous pathologist who discovered leukaemia, abominated Bismarck and relaid the Berlin drains. Virchow looked down his microscope and pronounced no cancer. Mackenzie cancelled the operation and went home.

His patient followed in June, for three months' Jubilee celebrations. Mackenzie continued to pick away at his larynx with forceps, as a bird at a nut. On 7 September, Queen Victoria summoned Mackenzie to Balmoral and knighted him in the drawing room after lunch.

The Crown Prince wintered among the flowers and palms of San Remo on the Italian Riviera. On 5 November, Mackenzie had a telegraphed summons to the Villa Zirio. The lump had grown frighteningly, spreading to the opposite vocal chord. 'Is it cancer?' asked the Crown Prince, in his whisper. Mackenzie answered, 'I am sorry to say, sir, it looks very much like it.' He had in May clumsily plucked a speck of normal tissue for Professor Virchow. Frederick gave a sad smile. 'Under the circumstances I really must apologize for feeling so well.'

The relations of doctors and the press were simple in the 1880s. You told the scoundrels nothing. The outraged German papers had blazed all summer at the Crown Princess for thrusting an English doctor against a future German

Emperor's sickbed (wrongly, but Viki's estimation of German medicine lay in every glance at her son's withered arm). San Remo was full of reporters, ambushing Mackenzie and training telescopes on the villa. The thunder of *The Times* rolled across the Channel.

The doctors started quarrelling with Mackenzie more openly than with each other. They became a round dozen with the arrival of Professor von Schrötter from Vienna, Dr Krause from Berlin and Dr Mark Hovell from Golden Square. Unlucky thirteen was Dr Moritz Schmidt, hurried from Frankfurt by Prince William, who had decided to take charge of the case himself.

William paraded the doctors. How long had his father to live? Eighteen months, said Mackenzie. How long had the cancer been there? Dr Krause volunteered, six months. 'I thought Mackenzie would die of shame!' exclaimed the future Kaiser. 'But his face, which I was watching narrowly, showed no trace of emotion.'

His mother disagreed. 'I cannot enough repeat how wise and kind, how delicate and considerate and judicious Sir Morell Mackenzie is,' she wrote to Queen Victoria. Her husband faced his doctors' alternatives. He could have his whole larynx excised immediately, which was more likely to be an assassination attempt than an operation. Or he could have a simple tracheostomy hole to breathe through, whenever necessary in the indefinite future. He chose the second. He was the calmest man in the room.

The press would be left in a mist, from which the hard facts could emerge gradually. The public grew as petulant as children kept from adults' secrets. William made the doctors sign a confidential bulletin admitting the truth, which in a couple of days leaked into the Berlin papers. In Berlin coffee houses they recalled the Salic Law, forbidding succession to the throne through the female line – Queen Victoria would otherwise have been also Queen of Hanover. The Hohenzollern family were muttered to have a similar rule, excluding the weakling and the sickly. Bismarck already had the doddery Emperor authorize young William to sign state papers in his father's stead, and planned to proclaim him Regent on his grandfather's death.

The gentle patient gently got worse. At 3 p.m. on 9 January 1888, the operation plotted the previous May was performed in the Villa Zirio's drawing room by a young Dr Bramann, who was experienced in tracheostomies for children choking with diptheria. Mackenzie issued a statement to the *Lancet* saying the disease was not cancer. Well, probably not. His daughter Ethel came from London and inflamed the German newspapers by playing tennis with Viki's daughter, particularly as they had discovered Mackenzie to be really a Polish Jew called Moritz Marcovicz.

The patient's strength declined. The doctors' increased. Professors Kaussmaul and Waldeyer made sixteen. On 9 March, the old Emperor William I died. The voiceless new one Frederick II took train through the Alpine snowstorms to Berlin. Everyone said that Bismarck arranged it, hoping the journey would kill him.

April 12 was a terrible afternoon. The tracheostomy hole Frederick breathed through needed a curved metal tube inside. Mackenzie was inserting a better design, and thought it tactful to invite Professor von Bergmann to the Neue Palais from Berlin. The galloping messenger traced him to a hotel. He was drunk. (He had pinned the aristocratic 'von' to his name. He was no Prussian, but a Slav from Riga, where they were notorious martyrs to the bottle.) He insisted on operating himself. He poked the tube into the neck muscles. The patient went blue. He followed it with his forefinger. The Emperor nearly died. The doctors scurrilously blamed each other, in private and the press. Queen Victoria arrived, and scolded Prince William for unfilial behaviour. Professor Leyden, Professor Senator, Dr Landgret and Professor Bardeleben of the Charité brought the medical squad to twenty. The Emperor started coughing up his own windpipe. After ninety-three days' reign, he died of bronchopneumonia.

The new Kaiser William II posted armed guards at all entrances and patrols of hussars in the grounds, forebade anyone to leave or send a telegram on pain of arrest, ransacked his father's private papers. Viki begged in tears that her husband be spared the defilement of a postmortem. William insisted. They sewed him up just in time for the lying-in-state. Overmanned to the last, he was anatomized by ten doctors.

Mackenzie left Germany with a £12,000 fee, the hate of the people and the spite of the press. The Kaiser and Bismarck accused him of deliberately concealing the diagnosis, that Frederick might escape being declared incapable of reigning. Perhaps they were right. Frederick had chosen at San Remo the unimpending risk, which promised brief rule to establish a government and reward politically slighted friends (Mackenzie got the Hohenzollern Cross and Star).

Bismarck's son, the Foreign Minister, asserted the Emperor would have lived for years without the misfortune of meeting Mackenzie. The German doctors castigated Mackenzie for stopping the May operation, which they wishfully insisted would have cured the disease. The German people more earthily accused him of ensuring the Empress's fatter pension for *die Engländerin*, who once possessed of her dowry was going to marry her chamberlain Count Seckendorff, everyone knew it for a fact.

Mackenzie retaliated. He sued *The Times* and the *St James's Gazette* for libel. In *The Fatal Illness of Frederick the Noble* he justified himself as Oliver Twist in a medical Fagin's kitchen. The book appeared in the lurid autumn of Jack the Ripper.

The public refused his dose of vitriol. Reviewers and editors were revolted by a quarrel over a corpse. The Royal College of Surgeons disparaged him for violating the secrets of the sick-room – as Lord Moran seventy-eight years later, after Churchill's deathbed. The Royal College of Physicians, whom Mackenzie had called 'an academy of decorous mediocracy', paid off old scores and made him resign. He stood amazed amid the shattered eggshell of his self-righteousness. He passed Whistler's presentation copy of

The Gentle Art of Making Enemies to his assistant – 'I do not seem to have any need to study it.' Two years later he was dead, aged fifty-four.

Mackenzie's expedition was a disaster, clinically, professionally and politically. The doctors applied to a disease of which they knew little treatment of which they should have been ashamed. It was an unusual case. The cancer supervened on another condition.

In 1888, *Drame Impérial* was published by Jean de Bonnefon, who had covered San Marino for the Paris newspaper *Gaulois*. He asserted that the Crown Prince had syphilis. He had caught it from a delicious *señorita* Dolores Cada. She was part of the celebrations at opening the Suez Canal in 1869. The Khedive's physician treated him sketchily, and Frederick returned to the tedium of being a dutiful husband. *Mais le germe n'etait pas mort il dormait.* Not dead, but sleepeth. When Mackenzie told Viki the correct diagnosis, she slapped his face.

The doctors at San Remo gave anti-syphilitic treatment with potassium iodide, soon gleefully discovered by the French papers. Mackenzie explained forcefully it was prescribed only *to exclude* – no cure, no syphilis. Professor von Schrötter scoffed at an *altes Weibergeschwätz*, old wives' tale.

Frederick was certainly syphilitic. A throat surgeon I knew as a houseman learned the secret from Mackenzie's most intimate friend. Mackenzie's reputation was attacked for what he did not say – that the Emperor had cancer. He suffered from what Mackenzie could not say – that the Emperor had syphilis.

No Victorian doctor could have saved Frederick. Had God not pressed His cancerous thumbprint for another ten years, perhaps democracy would have rooted in Germany, the mighty German Army and magnificent British fleet peacefully policed the world, Kaiser William grown to wiser ways. Instead, Queen Victoria died in the Kaiser's arms, and threequarters of a million of her countrymen in his defiance.

15

The Tender Trap
Delicate disaster

The solution for male doctors who do rough pelvic exams on women might begin in medical schools, where each male student would be placed in stirrups and a strange female MD would come and 'squeeze his balls and leave without saying a word'. That's the advice of Dr Joan Magee, a gynaecologist, writing in the *Annals of Internal Medicine*.

Chatelaine Magazine

16

Scutari
Miss Nightingale v. *the British Army*

The things they say about Florence Nightingale.

'She was a shocking nurse,' affirmed her sister Parthenope, who had felt her relentless touch. She was not a ministering angel, but a resolute administrator and ruthless politician. She did not sail for the Crimea with dedicated high-born ladies, but a mixture of agitated nuns and ginny Sarah Gamps.

She was named because her mother happened to be staying at Florence on the Italian tour. She could as easily have been called Leghorn. The lamp on her statue in Pall Mall and illuminating our £10 note is wrong. She carried a linen Turkish lamp like a Chinese lantern. The soldiers were supposed to kiss her shadow. I have been in the dark with a nurse and the lamp at Miss Nightingale's St Thomas's Hospital, and it does not throw light enough to kiss anything.

Britain has dispatched admirals on hazardous missions from Cadiz to the Falklands, and needed shoot only one on his own quarterdeck. The Crimea was a disaster because the British Army was still mentally fighting Waterloo – forty-nine years before, when medical supplies were a luxury and soldiers' welfare a fantasy.

The four-towered Selinie Quicklaci barracks beside the vast Scutari cemetery – still seen across the Bosphorus like a massive upturned billiards table – was made a hospital by whitewashing the walls. There were no bandages or bedpans, mattresses or mugs, food or fuel. Constantinople lying far farther south than Bournemouth was assumed in London to be hot.

They had plenty of rats and lice, and 250 soldiers' wives and widows getting drunk and prostituting themselves in the basement. They had some wooden operating tables, but chopped them up for firewood. In the bitter November of 1854, Miss Nightingale and 1050 casualties from the Charge of the Light Brigade arrived simultaneously.

The army doctor in charge of Scutari was across the Black Sea at Balaklava – Dr John Hall, who forbàde chloroform because 'the smart of the knife is a powerful stimulant, and it is better to hear a man bawl lustily than to see him sink silently into his grave'. The only nurses were soldiers unfit for anything else. Medical stores from home were labelled 'Not Urgent', and the *Prince* bringing them sailed first to the Crimea, where she sank in a hurricane.

The wounded, packed on the transports from the Crimea to Turkey, had abandoned their knapsacks in the summer's forced march on the Alma; they possessed only filthy greatcoats as blankets on deck, suffered frostbite, dysentery, typhus, scurvy and cholera, and went overboard dead at a dozen a day. At Scutari, the daily rate from four miles of patients lining its floors was forty-five. The stench penetrated the walls. As Bernard Shaw mentioned, 'The

British soldier can stand up to anything except the British War Office.'

Miss Nightingale was crammed into the 'Sisters' Tower' (found to contain a dead Russian general), with forty nurses on 12*s* a week (double London pay), in hideous uniforms (to repel the men), and allowed to drink gin (in moderation). She could not enter a ward without an army doctor's order. The army preferred to ignore her. The nurses sewed idly. But Miss Nightingale had a way of getting her way. 'I MUST remember God is not my private secretary,' she once wrote a note to herself.

Florence Nightingale had a rich, idle father, a fashionable matchmaking mother and a flower-arranging sister. She was thirty-four, had confessed the nursing urge ten years before to Julia Ward Howe, the American suffragist. Her family were perplexed and disgusted. A nurse was lower socially than the maid who emptied their slop-buckets. The Institution for the Care of Sick Gentlewomen in Distressed Circumstances in Harley Street timorously appointed her superintendent, driving her mother to sal volatile, her sister to bed for a week and her father to the Athenæum Club.

She installed within months windlass lifts for the food, piped hot water and a bleeping system with bells, banned the crinoline, killed the vermin, fired the house-surgeon, cut up the worn chaircovers for dishcloths, bulk-ordered the groceries from Fortnum and Mason's, made her own jam at tuppence a pot, took a patients' library subscription at Mudie's, and reduced the daily cost of each inmate from 1*s* 10*d* to 1*s*. She embodied the no-nonsense, down-to-earth, roll-up-the-sleeves approach to the, agonies of the body, mind and heart which is the glory of the Englishwoman. She would have been equally efficient running Dartmoor Gaol and probably as happy.

The Sick Gentlewomen were valuable guineapigs for the sick soldier. Next year at Scutari she swabbed the wards, emptied the overflowing latrine tubs, scoured the drains (producing 2 dead horses, 24 assorted animals and 556 handcarts of rubbish), stuffed straw in bags for beds, found cauldrons to heat the water, set the soldiers' wives scrubbing and washing, raided the quartermaster's stores, broke all regulations and defied everybody, knowing she could never be court-martialled.

Miss Nightingale had two priceless allies. William Howard Russell's chilling dispatches had crystallized national fury. His *Times* raised £30,000 for her purse in the bazaars of Constantinople, to buy knives and forks, soap and towels, food and drink, bedding and clothing – you were nursed in what you were wounded in. The British ambassador was baffled at her rejecting his suggestion of using the money to raise British prestige by erecting a Protestant church.

M. Alexis Soyer, famous chef of the Reform Club, as exuberantly French as only one who has lived all his life in London, left for Scutari on an impulse over scalloped oysters and port in Drury Lane. He redeployed the kitchens and drilled the cooks, applied intelligence and flavouring to the salt meat, sheep heads, cow heels and offal, turned the inedible into the desirable. The men cheered him in the wards. 'Though admittedly it has no nourishing qualities, there is nothing yet discovered which is substitute to the English for . . .' Ah! Miss Nightingale! Your genius for essentials! '. . . his cup of tea.'

'The Bird' claimed justly to have started nursing the British Army, then clothing it, feeding it, writing its letters home, making its wills and burying a good proportion of it. 'Nursing is the least of the functions into which I have been forced.' She had plenty of dirty women to do the dirty work.

Miss Nightingale presided that winter at 2000 deathbeds. The mortality rate fell to 5 per cent in the spring. The last patient left in summer the following year. She had been at war for 632 days and came home with a reputation for life. She went to bed for fifty years. From her Mayfair couch she reorganized the Army Medical Department, sanitated India, founded her nurses' training school, wrote *Notes on Nursing* and *Suggestions for Thought to the Searchers*

after Truth among the Artizans of England, to which Mr John
Stuart Mill was most kind. Cabinet ministers, generals,
viceroys entered her bedroom beseeching advice, Master
of Balliol Jowett that she should marry him. It was an age
when women's liberation meant going without stays. They
gave her the Order of Merit and she died, aged ninety.

Miss Nightingale revolutionized nursing by making a
chambermaid's work an occupation for gentlewomen. Her
system was so sound that her antiseptic ghost haunts every
sickbed. Wherever you are ill, you are still nursed by Florence Nightingale.

She was a woman of whom our country is rightly proud,
because she could not possibly have come from any other.

17

The Most Unkindest Cut of All

Vasectomy vagaries

I have treated no patients for thirty years, but am regularly
solicited for medical advice at parties and picnics, across
dinner tables and bars, and by people overhearing me
called 'Doctor' in the queue at the bank or the butcher's.
Once signing my works in a classy London bookshop, I
was interrupted by a clergyman pulling up his sombre
trouser leg and inviting inspection of his knee. He explained
you had to wait so long in the surgery. Perhaps patients
prefer consulting me, because any disagreeable advice carries no moral obligation of its acceptance, or even belief.

One case I can diagnose on its approach with vodka and
tonic in hand. A man under thirty with a low-handicap
look, who volunteers that the two kids are fine, but they're
changing the Datsun for a Volvo and its Florida this summer, not Ibiza, and there's all this in the papers about the
pill, why not end the fretting and fussing at a stroke, well

two strokes, I'm thinking seriously about a vasectomy, Doc, what would you advise me to do?

Vasectomy is the securest contraceptive next to abstinence. Sterilization knows no equality – the failure rate is 0·02 per cent for men, 0·13 per cent for women. The pill has a failure rate of 0·16 per cent, intra-uterine devices of 1·5 per cent, foaming chemicals of 11·9 per cent, the condom of 3·6 per cent, coitus interruptus of 6·7 per cent and the rhythm method a discordant 15·5 per cent.

A vasectomy is also a declaration of marital adherence more solemn than anything uttered at the altar.

The cut lifeline is the vas deferens, a muscular-walled tube conveying sperm from the testicle to the world at large. It runs through hernia country. The surgeon can feel a hard thread among the small arteries, veins and nerves composing the spermatic cord. These strands are wrapped in the filmy cremaster muscle, performer of the cremasteric reflex, a tautening on the testes in response to someone delicately stroking the inner thigh. This is more agreeable, if the circumstances are right, to having your knee-jerks hammered.

Vasectomy is as fashionable an ingredient of active, modern male life as skin-diving, windsurfing and hang-gliding. It was being performed in the days of hansom cabs and the bustle. 'This treatment is already obsolescent,' the *Theory and Practice of Surgery* dismissed the operation in 1903. They tried it to shrink enlarged prostates, but the patients 'have rapidly aged or become demented from this loss, it has been conjectured, of the stimulating influence of testicular secretion'. In the 1930s it was done for rejuvenation, in the 1940s to prevent infection after prostate surgery.

The operation is performed under local. The patient needs only spare an hour from his day and spend longer than usual shaving that morning. Like all operations, it is more difficult than it looks. Each spermatic cord is exposed at the root of the penis, a slice of vas deferens cut, the ends sealed. Both sections go under the laboratory microscope. The surgeon may snip vein or tendonous muscle by mistake, disastrous when the patient revels in his new freedom (the record is two hours post-operatively, including lunch in Soho). Insisting the patient has a sperm count before letting fly avoids the surgeon being sued for making his wife pregnant.

The vasectomized virgin dons a tie invitingly lettered IOFB – I Only Fire Blanks. Intact males retaliate with IFLR, more puzzling and equally vulgar.

Vasectomy guillotines a man's reproductive life thirty years before its death from natural enfeeblement. The young husband resuming the nuptial couch, as incapable of fatherhood as a mysogynic eunuch, may later wish to change this piece of bedroom furniture. His joyful ability to plant without reaping may encourage it, in widening the circle of his feminine acquaintances. The stark new marriage demands the embellishment of children. He returns to his surgeon.

Restoring a vasectomy is more difficult than taping together plastic garden hose chewed by the dog. The fiddly operation of vaso-vasotomy may not work. It is unfortunate that we cannot install a stopcock. Perhaps the solution is bottling some sperm pre-vasectomy, and laying it down in the deep freeze for enjoyment several years later, like home cooking.

My good friend and neighbour, distinguished doctor-writer David Delvin, wrote up his own vasectomy in the late seventies. As a moving example of self-sought tragedy it matches *Othello*.

The post-operative morning, disaster struck. The ligature slipped from his spermatic artery. What Australians call the family jewel box began to swell. Within minutes, it resembled a coconut. Within hours, it matched a honey-dew melon. By nightfall, it was indistinguishable from a football. By morning, the colour deepened and it could have passed for a city gentleman's bowler hat.

The disabled doctor could reach the telephone across the room only on all fours, suspending the afflicted parts with a squash-racket clutched beneath his breastbone. When young men at parties now cadge advice about vasectomy, I simply clap them on the shoulder and bark, 'Buy a squash-racket!'

18

Bitter Victory

Spanish flu

At the eleventh hour, the eleventh day in the eleventh month, the killing stopped. The world rejoiced, the gods laughed.

The Great War killed 8,538,313 military personnel, 12·5 per cent of the 65,038,810 mobilized. The influenza pandemic of 1918 killed 0·5 per cent of the entire population of the United States and of England, 3 per cent of Sierra Leone's, 25 per cent of Samoa's and 60 per cent of the Eskimos in Nome, Alaska. In six weeks it killed 3·1 per cent of US recruits at Camp Sherman. Five million died in India, often untidily – the corpses needed removing from overcrowded trains on arrival. Liners docked with 5 per cent fewer passengers than embarked.

The big American push on the Meuse-Argonne front was checked by 70,000 flu casualties. So was Ludendorff's last fling on the Somme. Woodrow Wilson got it, also Lloyd George, Clemenceau, German prime minister Prince Max and Colonel House.

Nature is a more efficient murderer than man. The war needed four years, the flu barely one. It killed 25,000,000, 3 per cent of all cases, our worst plague. A fifth of the global population caught it, it left serological fingerprints on many more who nursed subclinical attacks.

Flu fatalities usually lie in infancy and senility. This epidemic mocked the war by slaughtering the 20–40 age group. Influenza was the tiger, pneumonia the jackal for its unkilled prey. Antibiotics lay as far ahead as Chancellor Hitler.

Where had it come from? The milder first wave started in US military camps during the spring of 1918, to be transported with the troops to France. Thence to Spain, where the fright was so violent the disease found its name. There was influenza that spring in China, and Chinese labourers mingled with men from everywhere crowded into Europe, coughing over each other.

A deadlier wave broke in the autumn, perhaps starting at Ashkhabad in southern Russia, crossing the Iranian border for an outbreak at Mashhad, in the corner against Afghanistan. That August, HMS *Africa* had sailed from Sierra Leone, losing 7 per cent of her crew before reaching the Channel. Like a malign Puck, infection girdled the earth with simultaneous outbreaks in the ports of Freetown, Brest and Boston. In the US it killed more new immigrants from rural Italy, Russia, Austria and Poland than from crowded Britain and Germany.

As Boccaccio said of an earlier scourge, 'How many valiant men, how many fair ladies, breakfasted with their kinsfolk and that same night supped with their ancestors in the other world.' People eyed each other with keener suspicion than during the war's spy scares. To sneeze was like drawing a knife. 'Coughing, Sneezing or Spitting Will not be Permitted in the Theatre,' said the notices outside. 'In case you must Cough or Sneeze, do so in your own handkerchief, and if the Coughing or Sneezing Persists Leave the Theatre At Once. *Go Home and Go to Bed until You Are Well.* If you have a cold or are coughing and sneezing *Do Not Enter This Theatre.*'

Hospitals had patients in the corridors. Thousands were inoculated with useless anti-flu vaccine. Schools and libraries were closed. Men were advised to stop shaves in barbershops. Everyone was advised to wear fresh pyjamas, avoid shaking hands, take castor oil. The world wore white cotton masks, like surgeons'. In San Francisco they were obligatory, on pain of gaol (the police complained they encouraged robbery).

Soldiers prudently dug graves for which there were not yet bodies. There was profiteering in coffins. The Washington DC health commissioner commandeered two railroad cars full of them, which a railwayman tipped him off to be lying in the Potomac freight yards. He stacked them under police guard, coffin theft being the crime of the moment.

The visitation lingered everywhere about six weeks. A less lethal wave came with 1919. By the spring, the flu had gone. Where? Perhaps into swine.

It could come back.

19

St Anthony's Fire
Bakehouse disaster

On 15 August 1951 the Provençal village of Pont Saint Esprit went mad.

One in twenty of its 4000 inhabitants were seized with delirium and hallucinations, ran wild in the streets, writhed and screamed in their beds, suffered nausea, colic, vomiting, insomnia and burning sensations, particularly in the anus. Four died.

It was St Anthony's fire, *ignis sacer, mal des ardents*, scourge of the medieval peasantry. You feel you are being burned at the stake. Your fingers and toes, hands and feet drop off. If doubly unlucky you have convulsions (it depends on your level of vitamin A).

The cause is bread milled from 'smutty' rye infected with ergot fungus (*Claviceps purpurea*), as anyone would tell you in the seventeenth century. The ergot grows purple spurs on the ears of rye, particularly after a wet sowing and a wet summer.

Thucydides' Plague of Athens was really ergot poisoning. It was uninfectious – no other Athenian cities got it. The symptoms were too varied for any single disease, and the naval expedition to Laconia suffered after loading supplies there. The cause was damaged crops salvaged from Attica.

The English had little taste for rye bread and little ergotism, apart from *A Singular Calamity, Which Suddenly Happened to a poor Family of this Parish, Of which Six Persons lost their Feet by a Mortification not to be accounted for,* perpetuated by a 1762 tablet in Wattisham village church, Suffolk.

Ergot contains an LSD-like chemical found also in morning glory seeds, everyday hallucinogen of the Aztecs. As drugs account for peculiar behaviour today, so bread in the Middle Ages. The eleven girl accusers in the Salem witchcraft trials of 1692 – who suffered 'distempers' of odd speech, postures and gestures, and fits – may have achieved the hanging of nineteen fellow creatures, and the pressing to death of another, while high on ergot.

Perhaps Aldous Huxley's seventeen orgiastic nuns possessed by the devils of Loudun – whose *furor uterinus* had priest Grandier truly burned at the stake – defeated their energetic exorcists because they were only coming through the rye.

20

Beachy Head

Preventive medicine breakthrough

The South Downs fall into the English Channel at Beachy Head, a sheer cliff 532 feet high, pure chalk, gleaming in the sun like an actress's smile.

To the east nestles the seemly Sussex resort of Eastbourne, largely owned by the Duke of Devonshire. Its small white hotels edge a Marine Parade on which pale wizened people sit in deck chairs reading Agatha Christie – the

population sinks to the bottom of Britain with passing
years, like the sand in an hour glass, in the pathetic hope
that the weather might be a little better. The Bell Tout
lighthouse was built atop the Head in 1831. The British
and Dutch fleet were beaten there by the French on 30
June 1690, our admiral the Earl of Torrington court-martialled for his pains.

What the Bernese Oberland is to serious skiers, Beachy
Head is to resolute suicides.

People were falling over Beachy Head before St Augus-
tine arrived along the coast at Thanet to convert the
Anglo-Saxons in 596. Two or three a year dropped off this
century, reaching a steady average of four in 1965. Like
other well-publicized open-air activities, the participants
recently steadily increased. In 1971 ten went over, in 1976
sixteen, in 1979 twelve.

You can commit suicide by diving head first from your
bedroom window. If choosing 532 feet gives the oppor-
tunity of changing your mind while in transit, there is
nothing you can do about it. The disastrous fascination of
Beachy Head as a springboard for shuffling off this mortal
coil is complex.

British Rail runs an excellent hourly service from London's Victoria Station, and the expense of a return ticket
is avoided. (Three out of four suicidal tumblers down the
cliffs travel from inland Britain, five in the last twenty years
came specially from abroad to do it.) Jumping off Beachy
Head runs in some families. One suicide generally brings
the next within a fortnight, another example of man's infinite suggestibility and lack of originality.

The most popular months are July and August (nineteen
each in fifteen years), March and June (thirteen). April is
the cruellest month nationally for self-destruction, but
drops only three people down Beachy Head. Friday is the
favourite day, indicating that not everybody lives for the
weekend. The busiest spot is by the new undercliff lighthouse (twenty-three in fifteen years). The White Cliffs of

Dover had only one suicide a year, but the summer bus schedules up Beachy Head are better.

Not everyone you see hurtling from Beachy Head is committing suicide. Cliffs are dangerous places for romping, bird-nesting, seeking sexual seclusion. There are accepted indications that the fall was intentional – a woman wandering away from her handbag, a man neatly folding his overcoat, or gulping a bottle of whisky, or shouting to look out down below, or making a graceful swallow dive. One taxi driver reflected too late on the fare who directed him there from the gates of a psychiatric hospital.

The grisly record of *felo de se* has brilliantly been stayed. Since 1975 the suicide rate at Beachy Head has been halved. This was achieved with no elaborate construction work, no complicated surveillance, and at no additional public expense. They changed the local coroner.

Like any judge or doctor, the coroner must dutifully, even fearlessly, say how the facts strike him. The new man needed far stronger persuasion that his subjects intended to topple over the grassy edge. The whisky drinkers enjoyed the benefit of being in no condition to decide clearly one way or another. From twenty Beachy Head deaths in 1965–9, 65 per cent were suicides. From sixty-five deaths in 1975–9, only 32 per cent were, a drop in ten years of 33 per cent.

This is a sensational advance in preventive medicine. Deaths from cancer had meanwhile *increased* by some 10 per cent, from heart disease by 5 per cent. A comparable triumph was the elimination of polio by prophylaxis with Salk vaccine.

Happily for mankind, the Beachy Head principle is being adapted to wider medicine. Any cause of death is a matter of honest opinion. The Royal College of Physicians of London claim that one-fifth of British death certificates give an incorrect reason, and a quarter contain other errors. Birmingham and Edinburgh, more advanced in research, have achieved a 40 per cent inaccuracy.

This method has already eradicated cholera from several

small tropical nations, putting it down as death from summer diarrhoea. In the distant, icy winter of 1939, medical officers prevented a humiliating epidemic of German measles in the British Army by reporting it as spots with a bad cold. The frightening new diseases which pour from research wards – Marfan's disease, Marchiafava–Michaeli syndrome, anti-glomerular basement membrane antibody nephritis, and the like – will thankfully be swiftly eliminated, because those family doctors who have heard of them will anyway be incapable of recognizing them.

Most people die in hospital from the Beachy Head syndrome. Elderly patients have so many diseases, the houseman puzzles which to put first. If he mentions the fall from a bicycle which brought the patient to the hospital six months ago, there will be endless fuss with the coroner. If he mentions 'alcoholism' he will outrage the relatives. If he mentions 'postoperative shock' he will outrage the surgeon. If he seeks advice, consultants are as unexcited about their dead patients as actors about their closed shows.

After playing the diagnoses like patience, the houseman generally selects bronchopneumonia – 'the old man's friend' of pre-antibiotic medicine – signs the death certificate and collects his ash cash (extra fee for cremation). It is a kindly laxity to diagnose to the dying only diseases so familiarly lethal. The patients can succumb to them in saintly resignation.

21

The King is Dead

Not without help

On the Sunday evening of 1 February 1685, Protestant King Charles II of England, aged fifty-three, sat fondling the Duchesses of Portsmouth, Cleveland and Mazarin – three of his thirteen mistresses – while a score of his courtiers crouched over a heap of two thousand golden guineas playing basset, a simple game depending on the turn of a card, and a French boy sang love songs.

At eight o'clock the next morning, just out of bed to be shaved, the King uttered a cry and had fits. Dr Edmund King, a guest at Whitehall Palace, applied emergency treatment by letting sixteen ounces of blood from a vein in the left arm, while messengers were sent galloping for the royal physicians.

The fashionable doctor was becoming the man of fashion – buckskin breeches and silver-buckled shoes, velvet coat and full-bottomed wig, tricorn hat and beaver muff in winter. His essential equipment was a gold-headed cane, its perforated head crammed with aromatic herbs to ward off infection, or at least the stink. The King paid his doctors £100 a year, and they charged half a guinea for coffee-house consultations. Bleeding a lady in bed cost 10*s*, a man half a crown, and you could get a postmortem for 3*s* 4*d*.

Everyday illness meant plague, typhus, smallpox. Surgery was setting limbs and cutting for stone. The doctors of Europe were restive for new ideas. Harvey had changed the heart from the seat of emotion to a pump (Dr Jonathan Miller says because pumps were proliferating with the thriving of mining). The Dutch had anatomized and microscoped. At Oxford, they were sniffing the vitality of oxygen. Health and disease were losing their mystique and becoming as worldly as profit and loss in a City of London counting house.

Was the body a machine, its teeth scissors, chest bellows, stomach grinding millstones? Or a vat of fermenting juices, to be blended skilfully by the doctors as the brewer his beer? These new philosophies were both shot through with immutable superstition. Molière did nicely out of it.

Treatment Fit for a King

MONDAY
Their leader Sir Charles Scarburgh said the six physicians 'Flocked quickly to the King's assistance; and after they

had held a consultation together, they strenuously endeavoured to afford timely succour to His Majesty in his dangerous state.'

Immediately they applied to his shoulders three cupping glasses like wine glasses, flamed to expel the air and raise mounds of skin. This treatment was performed in the Stone Age with animals' horns. Cupping was instantly followed by scarification, for eight ounces of blood.

'Within a few moments of this,' recounted Sir Charles, 'so as to free his stomach of all impurities, and by the same action to rid his whole nervous system of anything harmful to it, we administered an Emetic.' This was antimony in the equivalent of curaçao, but the King jibbed. They gave him vitriol in peony water, a couple of purgative pills and the clyster.

It was the golden age of the clyster, delivered through the nozzle of a metal syringe, as used for spraying roses. Application and result was such a beautiful demonstration of Descartes' *l'homme-machine*.

'Wind doth now and then torment me about the fundament extremely,' complained Pepys, whose wife ministered him one of strong ale, four ounces of sugar and two ounces of butter. ('Two stools in the night – pissed well.')

The King's was less robustly tasty – mallow leaves, violets, beet, camomile flowers, fennel seeds, linseed, cinnamon, cardamom, saffron, cochineal and aloes. It was repeated after two hours, accompanied orally with syrup of blackthorn, more antimony and some rock salt.

The physicians were impatient. They dropped another charge of purgatives, shaved his hair and stuck blistering plasters all over his head. The King had more fits. They sent for the red-hot cautery.

Before its arrival, the King luckily regained consciousness. The doctors were ecstatic. How brilliantly their treatment worked! The patient must enjoy more of it.

To relieve the pressure of humours, they purged as a matter of course and excited sneezing with white hellebore root up the nostrils. They gave powdered cowslip flowers to strengthen the brain, then more purgatives to keep the bowels going during the night. The blistering plasters of cantharidin – 'Spanish fly', the ageless aphrodisiac – irritated the urinary passages when absorbed through the skin and excreted. The doctors treated scalding urine with a soothing decoction of barley, licorice and sweet almond kernels. The King's supper was thin broth and ale without hops. They plastered the soles of his feet with tar and pigeon dung, gave him another enema and said goodnight.

TUESDAY

The patient was *much* better! 'The blessing of God being approved by the application of proper and seasonable remedies,' Sir Charles congratulated the Almighty and himself. They told the King to go on taking the potions.

The doctors were now twelve. This treatment of royalty by committee – persisting disastrously for Frederick of Prussia two hundred years later – is ruthlessly rich in bright suggestions. At noon, they opened both jugulars for ten ounces of blood. They gave a gargle of elm in syrup of mallow for his sore throat. To prevent more fits, they prescribed a julep of black cherry, peony, lavender, crushed pearls and white sugar candy, which sounds lovely.

WEDNESDAY

The doctors' sunny confidence brought milder draughts of senna pods infused in spring water, given with white wine and nutmeg. At five that afternoon, they issued their first bulletin from the Whitehall Council Chamber for the morrow's *London Gazette*, ending, 'That they conceive His Majesty to be in a condition of safety, and that he will in a few days to be freed from his distemper.'

THURSDAY

When the bulletin appeared, the King was nearly dead. He suddenly had more fits. During the night they gave him spiritous draught of skull from a man meeting violent death, the clinical equivalent of extreme unction.

74

The King's ministers grew anxious and angry. What was His Majesty suffering *from*? The doctors had no idea.

They consulted urgently. Intermittent fever! There was a lot of it about in London that time of year. And they could cure it! Send for the Peruvian bark, quick!

This was chincona bark, full of quinine. It was picturesquely named after the Countess of Chinchon, wife to the Spanish Viceroy of Peru, well known to be miraculously cured of malaria by it (in fact, she died of something else in Cartagena, still on her way to Peru). 'Jesuits' bark' was being dispensed by the Society of Jesus in Lima in the 1630s, and Oliver Cromwell could hardly swallow it.

They gave it three-hourly in milk, interspersed with more human skull.

Neither worked.

FRIDAY

The King was worse. That night, they had to use Raleigh's Stronger Antidote and Goa Stone. He apologized for being an unconscionable time dying and asked them not to let poor Nelly starve. Towards dawn, they gave the Oriental Bezoar Stone, a rare concretion from the stomach of an East Indian goat. The King grew breathless. He was bled. At 8.30 in the morning his speech faltered and failed. At ten he was comatose. At noon he died (as a Roman Catholic).

SATURDAY

The King was rumoured to have been poisoned. So were most at the time. A postmortem was held. The brain was engorged with blood, there was old pleurisy of the right lung, the heart was enlarged. Nothing else was wrong. The illness seemed hardly worth all the fuss.

Charles II probably died from high blood pressure, after kidney failure caused by his gout. The treatment neither delayed nor hastened his death, only made it more painful and wretched. His physicians were doing their best, according to their lights. Who dares claim our medical lights today always shine truer than will-o'-the-wisp?

22

Obstetrical Obsession
Maternal mutilation

A baby joyously enters the world much like a circus clown bursting head first through a paper hoop. The rips are immediately neatly stitched – gynaecologists enjoy the Biblical appellation of sewers of tears in other men's fields.

To snip with scissors the stretched perineum, against which the baby is lustily butting, had seemed for years an elegant stroke of preventive medicine. No one amid the bustle and alarms of maternity thought twice about it, until the National Childbirth Trust in 1981 called this operation of episiotomy, 'A genital mutilation, the most common form of genital mutilation we have in the West'.

The shocked comparison was to female circumcision, ceremonially performed in Central and East Africa on ten- to fourteen-year-old girls, one sweep of a sharp knife and white chicken feathers to dress the wound.

'Episiotomies are done much too casually and women are far too often teaching material for students,' objected the NCT lady. Of 1800 mothers studied, she discovered the two-thirds who suffered this unthinking obstetrical manoeuvre were twice as liable to severe pain the first week after delivery. More disastrously, many complained their sex lives were ruined for a year, causing marital disintegration.

This doomful diagnosis is contradicted by the oldest obstetrical story.

MIDWIFE: [*Visiting patient's home, surveying site of delivery five days afterwards*]. Now, Mrs Jones, I'm going to remove your episiotomy stitches – Mrs Jones! They've gone!

PATIENT: Oh, my husband took them out.
MIDWIFE: [*Horrified*] *Your husband took them out!*
PATIENT: Yes, Sister. He said they tickled.
  [*Collapse of stout nursing party*]
Unfortunately, NCT seems to have no sense of humour.

23

Sandwich Disaster

Botulism on Loch Maree

Loch Maree is formed in Wester Ross, Scotland, by the river Garry. This rises on Ben Lair ten miles to the south, and continues northwest between flat, heather-speckled banks as the river Ewe, gathering large burns running from the hill lochs. It flows into the Atlantic as Loch Ewe, opposite the north tip of Skye and the Outer Hebrides. It has fantastic seatrout.

Loch Maree is fifteen miles by three, with half a dozen small islands in the middle, cradled by mountains reaching three thousand feet. The countryside is Nature's plain gift, barely refined by the artful hand of man, which the Scots so cherish in their scenery and their cooking.

On Monday, 14 August 1922, the bracken was starting to crisp but the evenings were still long, if chilly – frost was recorded that midnight at Glasgow. The day was overcast and sprinkled with showers. The forty-four guests who filled the famed Loch Maree Hotel enjoyed 'a good, honest, wholesome, hungry breakfast' recommended by Izaak Walton, and split into fishing parties of two anglers in a boat, with a ghillie to row. Fishermen intending to make a day of it were furnished with half a dozen sandwiches – cold meat, chicken-and-ham paste, and wild duck potted meat – cut in the kitchen that morning.

The agreeable noonday moment arrived for unscrewing

the beer bottle, uncapping the hip flask, unwrapping the crinkly greaseproof paper. Major Anderson of the Seaforth Highlanders, on leave from India, preferred the cold beef. He passed the potted meat to his ghillie, though his wife Rosamund thought wild duck rather fun.

With the Great War barely four years dead, the holiday sparkled with rank. Brigadier-General Nichol found the potted meat nasty and lunched off cheese and biscuits. Colonel Lane finished his wild duck with relish. The gentlemen were so generous with sandwiches to the ghillies, young Ian Mackenzie could slip a selection into his creel for his wife.

The day's catch was weighed and laid in state on a marble slab in the hotel hall. The guests dressed and dined, to pass the evening with bridge and books. Before breakfast next morning, twenty-two-year-old John Talbot, just down from Oxford, holidaying with his barrister father and his mother, complained of seeing double. As the news spread through the dining room, John Stewart – he was big in wool at Paisley – exclaimed that he too suffered the curious condition. He was puzzled at an inability to remove one of the two baps on his plate. Everyone chortled. Seeing double? Been at the usquebaugh rather early in the day, old boy, eh what?

The two butts abandoned breakfast. They felt dizzy. Their eyelids began to droop. This was alarming. They felt tightening in the throat. They began to vomit and sweat. They staggered, had to lie down. Their speech became husky, indistinct, vanished. They could not swallow their spit. They could barely move arms and legs. They could hardly breathe. In his cottage along the Loch, ghillie Kenneth MacLennon was perplexed at his neighbour's smoking two pipes at once. Mrs Rosamund Anderson, Mrs Dixon from Dublin during the morning developed the same symptoms, by nightfall were dead. Mr Talbot and Mr Stewart died early next day. Brigadier-General Nichol and Colonel Lane felt fine.

The peaceful, pleasurable hotel held the horror of a

country-house, mass-murder mystery. The remoteness which the holidaymakers craved turned upon them terrifyingly. The nearest town was Gairloch, barely a thousand inhabitants, thirty miles from the railway, with no hospital nor telephone. The awesome double vision struck other trembling guests, the same symptoms ruthlessly followed, they went to their rooms and died.

Mrs Dixon's husband died on Thursday morning, ghillie MacLennon on Thursday night. On Monday, 21 August, went sixty-five-year-old Mr Willis, another barrister from London (accompanied by his valet). Ghillie Mackenzie was the last, late Monday night, leaving a young widow and two children. 'Happily, several medical men were staying in the hotel,' *The Times* looked on the bright side, 'and the sufferers had the best of care and attention.'

Front-page headlines announced 'Scottish Poison Mystery' and 'Deadly Paste Sandwiches'. *The Times* carried black-edged columns, but because of its owner Lord Northcliffe dying the same Monday (of syphilis, but nobody dared mention it).

The Loch Maree picnic captivated the public, like the equally inexplicable and chilling Loch Ness Monster ten years later. The eight deaths were vaguely attributed to 'ptomaine poisoning'. Botulism was first mentioned on the Friday by local Medical Officer of Health Dr Maclean, who had hurried cross-country from Dingwall by motorcar.

Botulism is not the food poisoning which ruins Mediterranean and Mexican holidays. It is a sudden, violent, paralysing nervous disease, caused by toxin from the germ *Clostridium botulinum*. The bacilli are short rods, which form resilient spores. They are scattered everywhere in the soil, useful in the decomposition of dead animals and plants. They grow only *without* oxygen – as in a jar of potted meat heated insufficiently in the factory to kill the spores. Sausages in Latin are *botuli*.

Botulinus toxin has the dangerous idiosyncrasy of acting when swallowed. To get tetanus from its brother *Clostridium tetani*, you have to cut yourself. Antitoxin treatment is unlikely to save life once symptoms appear. If you suffer double vision after potted meat, do not take a taxi to hospital, scream for an ambulance.

Loch Maree was the first outbreak of botulism in Britain. The previous outbreak in Europe was twenty-five years earlier, three Germans dying after eating ham. The last in America was only two months before, six dead in Idaho from home-canned vegetables. In the United States, home canning is more dangerous than home brewing. (Only fruit is safe, the acidity kills the bacillus.)

An inquiry under Scotland's Sudden Deaths Act was convened a fortnight later at Dingwall, Sheriff Mackintosh sitting with a jury. It emerged that the wild duck potted meat was bought from an Inverness grocer in June, a consignment of two dozen glass jars from Lazenby's of London (Est. 1795). Lazenby's had been potting duck in their Bermondsey factory for thirty-five years, 700 jars to the batch. They bought the wild duck in Leadenhall Poultry Market, just like the Savoy Hotel. Only one pot of the paste was infected.

Lazenby's dispatched north a King's Counsel with a watching brief. Dr Maclean revealed that he had just consumed, in the cause of truth and science, a tin of Maconachie's rations intended for the Boer War. Counsel asked, 'You suffered no ill effects?' 'Well, I am still here.' (*Laughter.*) It was a tragedy too baffling to take seriously.

Like the magistrate contemplating the death of young Albert Ramsbottom, eaten by the lion at Blackpool in Stanley 'Alfred Doolittle' Holloway's monologue, Sheriff Mackintosh comfortably 'gave his opinion that no one was really to blame'. If the jury was a generation ahead of its time in demanding 'sell by' dates on groceries, four of its seven were women.

The deadly jar must somehow have escaped sterilization in Bermondsey. It was a disaster for the canned food trade for years. Lloyd's of London offered hotels and boarding houses insurance against food poisoning, £1000 cover for half a crown a bed. A tin of Alaskan salmon as a treat for tea was as lethal fifty-six years later in the British Midlands. It cost the canners £2 million. In 1982, a Belgian died from salmon canned at Ketchycan, Alaska. The tear in a few tins, hidden by the label, necessitated the recall of five million others.

The same year, botulism struck the Thames, ravaging the swans. Luckily, it turned out to be the wrong diagnosis. It was lead poisoning from the anglers' weights.

Loch Maree was the only instance in history of Russian roulette played with sandwiches.

24

Breaking It Off

Liberated female disaster

Prolonged intercourse, particularly with the female subject in the superior position, and inadvertent flexion of the erect penis are well-described cases of penile trauma commonly leading to corporeal rupture.

Journal of Urology

25

101 Uses of a Dead Pope

Disaster on Judgement Day

After the appalling attack outside St Peter's on 13 May 1981, Pope John Paul II was rushed to the Gemelli Clinic, where Dr Giancarlo Castiglioni removed in a 4-hour 10-minute operation two bullets and the damaged sections of intestine.

The disposal of these scraps was more delicately circum-
spect than bits of ourselves, or of President Reagan in the
George Washington University Hospital six weeks earlier.

Tissue excised in the operating theatre is ordinarily
dropped into a stainless steel dish held by the scrub nurse,
tipped into a plastic sack and incinerated with the day's
debris. One Harley Street throat surgeon pocketed the
tonsils and adenoids, swearing they worked wonders on his
strawberry beds. But the Vicar of Christ must be rever-
enced, even in fragments.

His Holiness's pieces of gut were taken to the baroque
church of Santi Vincenzo ed Anastasio, opposite the Trevi
fountain. This was rebuilt in 1630, parish church of the
next door Palazzo del Quirinale. The crypt contains the
sacra praecordia. Here repose the entrails removed during
embalming of all popes from Sixtus V (died 27 August
1590). They are kept in large terracotta jars. The general
public is not admitted.

The praecordium is an everyday clinical term for the
area of chest over the heart. The Latin is anatomically
imprecise, meaning bowels, stomach, diaphragm. Eccle-
siastically it conveys 'the holy region before the heart' or
'the sacred internal organs'. The words carry a mystical
meaning beyond the workmanlike minds of those who every
day make 'no small presumption to dismember the image
of God' – as Queen Elizabeth's I's surgeon, John Woodall,
humbly recognized. Medically, a dead pope is no different
from a dead poacher.

The traumatized organs of our present vigorous Pope
must wait many years to be joined by their healthy fellows.
Three dozen popes have been embalmed since Sixtus V,
their entrails deposited in the Piazza di Trevi, their husks
borne to the Vatican Grottoes under St Peter's. When jolly
Pope John Paul I, who died after thirty-three days, was
kept too long above ground in a hot Roman September –
for his funeral to go out live during US TV prime time –
the deficiencies of a botched embalming job grew noisomely
noticeable.

Come Judgement Day, trunk and organs will be united
that a shining procession of popes may parade past the
seat of the Almighty. This is the well-publicized divine
plan for us all. But God made man in his image, which
suggests a celestial snafu when the Last Trump blows.
Judgement Day will be dreadfully confusing, with the jostling and the trumpets and the wails of the sinners, as
Michelangelo indicated with customary vision on the east
wall of the Sistine Chapel. The angelic reassembly of the
Holy Fathers will be a more distracted operation than the
slick mechanisms of Detroit.

'Michael,' comes the heavenly intercom a mile and a
half across Rome from the Piazza di Trevi to the Piazza
San Pietro. 'Can you help me, old man? I seem to have
got the right kidney of Clemens IX left over down here.'

'Gee, I'm sorry, Philip. But I guess I'm fully equipped
kidneywise over here.'

'But Mike, how *is* Clemens IX? I mean, does he look
like a pope with only one kidney?'

'Clemens looks fine, Phil, absolutely dinky. He's enjoying
his breakfast. Nothing like lying around since 1669 to give
a man an appetite.'

'Mike, old chap. Are you sure he *is* Clemens IX?'

'Recognize him anywhere, Phil.'

'I mean, you haven't got the wrong head on him?'

'Hey! Wait a minute. So I have! It's eating Benedict
XIII's eggs benedict. Fancy that, eh? I'll just move 'em
around . . . excuse me, Your Holiness. Thanks a lot. Say,
Phil?'

'Yes, Mike?'

'Got Innocent XI's left leg out there by any chance? You
could fly it in.'

'Sorry, Mike. Best I can do is Alexander VII's pancreas.
Are you sure, old chap, that Innocent XI had a left
leg?'

'Maybe there *was* a one-legged pope, Phil, but I've sure
never heard of one with three arms, like Leo XI at this
moment.'

'Look, be an angel and let me have Urban VIII back. Inside, he's Gregory XIV.'

I expect it will be all right on the Day.

26

Doctor Death

Nemesis on the down express

George Orwell dates the decline of the English murder from 1925, when the perfect crime for the Sunday papers was perpetuated by 'a little man of the professional class – a dentist or a solicitor, say – living an intensely respectable life somewhere in the suburbs, and preferably in a semi-detached house, which will allow the neighbours to hear suspicious sounds through the wall. . . . He should plan it all with the utmost cunning, and only slip up over some tiny unforseeable detail'.

Murderers, like garage mechanics, have lost love for their work. They shoot, knife, bludgeon and flee, instead of plotting with devilish ingenuity. Such carelessness does not mirror their relief from errors costing their life. Exceptional cleverness, infinite pains fail hopelessly to outwit the modern police laboratory.

This salutarily inhibiting science of forensic medicine was invented by Sir Bernard Spilsbury, of Oxford and St Mary's Hospital, London.

In 1910, Spilsbury examined 'the remains', dug from Dr Crippen's suburban cellar, identified them as Mrs Cora Crippen despite the lack of limbs, bones, genital organs and head (none ever found), and discovered them full of poisonous hyoscine. The literate world relished the torments of the down-at-heel doctor from Coldwater, Michigan, fleeing home across the Atlantic with his typist Ethel Le Neve disguised as a boy, 'trapped by wireless', overtaken by a Scotland Yard inspector in a fast liner, arrested in the St Lawrence river, brought home in handcuffs, tried in pomp at the Old Bailey. Thirty-three-year-old Spilsbury was like an unknown tenor making his name in a gala performance at Covent Garden.

He appeared with all the greats of murder in its greatest age.

In 1912, he was seen opposite Frederick Seddon, the London insurance agent who gave arsenic from fly-papers to his lady lodger for her £4000 life's savings. In 1915 with Brides-in-the-Bath specialist George Smith, who did for three of them under the taps. In 1922 with Herbert Armstrong, the churchwarden who poisoned his wife and was charged in the remote Welsh court where he sat as clerk – which had no lamps and needed to adjourn when daylight faded.

During 1924, Patrick Mahon cut Emily Kay into little bits, boiling some of her in a saucepan on the living-room fire, grinding the bones, scattering her all over his seaside bungalow at the Crumbles, near Beachy Head. Spilsbury caught the Eastbourne express from Victoria, fitted her together like a three-dimensional jigsaw, even found her two months pregnant. For the first time he gave the full service, including postmortem after execution.

Spilsbury shared the limelight with butcher Louis Voison, who put his mistress's torso in a sack labelled *Argentina La Plata Cold Storage* during a Zeppelin raid. Then with the famous duo Edith Thompson and Frederick Bywaters, a seafarer with the stylish P & O line, both hanged for knifing her husband in the East London suburb of Ilford (Spilsbury thought Edith was guiltless).

It was fashionable among murderers before World War Two to dismember their victims, pack them in trunks and leave them at railway stations. Mr Crossman cemented Mrs Crossman into a tin trunk in 1902, Mr Devereux dispatched his wife and twin children in similar luggage to a furniture depository in 1905. Nineteen twenty-seven brought the Charing Cross Station trunk murder (wicker-work trunk covered with black oilcloth), 1933 the first

Brighton one (plywood covered with brown canvas, legs in a suitcase at King's Cross), a month later the second Brighton one (black canvas). In 1935 no trunk, but legs and feet with corns under a carriage seat at Waterloo.

Spilsbury's hands were in all this baggage. The coincidence of trunks and torsos fascinates the public like beds and actresses. He rocketed to the popularity of Sherlock Holmes. (Murderers have gone off trunks. This is because of the international decrepitude of railways, and the fad for compact baggage necessitating a hard night's work with the Magimix.)

Spilsbury manipulated scalpel, microscope and test tube with dour thoroughness. To find the effect of a bullet through skin, he cadged an amputated leg from a surgeon and peppered it with a revolver. To test his theory on the brides in the bath, he had a St Mary's nurse volunteer for a tub (scientific accuracy assumedly precluding a swimsuit), ducking her with an unexpected tug of the legs. 'The nurse in question nearly died,' the Director of Public Prosecutions revealed later.

No case was buried with its victim. Spilsbury took the first train and dug it up.

When arsenic has closed your eyes,
This certain hope your corpse may rest in:
Sir B. will kindly analyse
The contents of your large intestine,

said *Punch* beneath his cartoon in rubber gloves and apron, wing collar and lavender spats.

He was tall and handsome, dressed by Savile Row, bowler-hatted by Lock of St James's, red carnation always in buttonhole. His shirt sleeves detached at the elbow, to save creasing the cuffs from repeated rolling up. All doctors develop a bedside manner, Spilsbury a dockside one. In the witness box he combined the assurance of God with the menace of the Devil. He was brief, clear, decisive, as untechnical as the medical columns of the picture papers. Juries loved him because they could understand him.

Judges the more so, because they needed not take the trouble to. He was ruffled only once, when insinuating his overwhelming medical authority to a junior barrister who responded, 'When did you last examine a *live* patient, Sir Bernard?'

A murder trial without Spilsbury was as unthinkable as *Cinderella* without the Fairy Godmother. His opinions were so impregnable he could achieve single-handed all the legal consequences of homicide – arrest, prosecution, conviction and final postmortem – requiring only the brief assistance of the hangman.

This reputation was perhaps as deterrent as the rope itself. A killer might think twice, aware of Spilsbury next morning sitting in a first-class carriage from London.

Or was it a reputation as deadly as the murderer boiling up his fly-papers, sharpening his cleaver, inquiring at Harrods for the luggage department?

Three months after Patrick Mahon was hanged for the Crumbles crime, Elsie Cameron was murdered by young Norman Thorne on a poultry farm twenty miles away across Sussex. He sawed her into four portions, crammed her head in a biscuit tin, wrapped the rest in sacking and buried her under his Leghorns. When taxed, he explained that she had arrived at his bungalow threatening to stay until he married her, he went out to the movies and came home to find her hanging from a beam. He cut her up in panic. So said Crippen about his Cora.

The police dug Elsie up for Spilsbury, forty-three days after death. The trial in the spring of 1926 occupied, like Mahon's, the beautiful county hall of Lewes. The wigs, the robes, the golden royal arms, the beautifully polished oak, the decorative judge, dignified counsel and decorous bobbies, afford an out-of-town murder trial the cosy charm of an English teaparty, with the incidental excitement that the guest of honour might be handed a poisoned cucumber sandwich.

Thorne's neck depended upon some marks on Elsie's. Spilsbury could find no signs of hanging, only the normal

skin creases. He thought she had been hit on the head and
strung up.

For the defence was pathologist Robert Brontë, a talk-
ative Irishman. He found the mark of a thin rope. So did
six other doctors. Spilsbury countered that Brontë had
examined the body forty-seven days after he did, for
twenty-eight of which it was buried in the London suburb
of Willesden, so not in prime condition. 'I have had over
twenty years' continuous experience of microscopic work
and the making of slides, applied more especially to medical–legal problems,' he crushed the court.

Elsie Cameron was a neurotic. Even balanced young
people impulsively kill themselves from frustrated passion.
Though it was seven to one against, the jury decided Dr
Brontë's evidence as imaginative as *Wuthering Heights*.

The prisoner was condemned; the press indicted Spilsbury. 'The unquestioning acceptance by the jury of Sir
Bernard Spilsbury's evidence . . . the singling out of this
particular medical witness for eulogy by the judge, seems
a legitimate point for comment.' The *Law Journal* objected
that the court 'followed the man with the biggest name'.
Conan Doyle was outraged. Perhaps he perceived like
Whistler that Nature was creeping up on his art.

Towards midnight on 23 October 1929, there was a fire
at the Metropole Hotel, Margate – a bleak and tawdry
resort on the Kent coast – in which sixty-three-year-old
Mrs Rosaline Fox was suffocated in her undervest. She was
staying there with her thirty-year-old son Sidney, in the
room next door. On 9 November, Spilsbury was on the
express from Liverpool Street Station to Norwich. Mrs Fox
was born in the Norfolk village of Great Frensham, where
she had been buried for ten days.

The coffin was sealed with putty, the body beautifully
fresh. Spilsbury found a bruise behind the larynx. A Margate doctor said she died from shock and suffocation, the
Margate coroner that hers was death by misadventure.
Spilsbury said it was by strangulation. Sidney Fox was
charged with murder. The case was transferred from Kent

to the same lovely courtroom in Lewes were Spilsbury and Brontë again confronted each other.

Brontë had seen no bruise. Spilsbury objected that Brontë got his hands on the body when putrefication made the bruise unrecognizable. Brontë responded that Spilsbury could not tell bruising from putrefaction. Fox was hanged.

That Fox was a swindler, a bilker of hotel bills, a flaunting homosexual, had been jailed for theft and forgery, had £3000 worth of insurance policies on his mother's life, all expiring that same midnight, was beside the point. He was hanged because a jury believed a bruise was there, simply because Spilsbury said so.

Like Noël Coward and the Duke of Windsor, Spilsbury did not fit comfortably into the world left by Hitler's war. At the Tottenham Court Road murder of April 1947 he was far from himself. His doctor son had been killed in an air raid, another died of TB. He suffered three strokes and from arthritis. On 17 December he performed a postmortem in Hampstead, dined at his club, and gassed himself in his laboratory in University College, Bloomsbury.

Spilsbury did 25,000 postmortems. About 250 of his subjects were murdered. If his evidence was wrong with only 3·3 per cent of them, his victims equalled Jack the Ripper's eight.

27

And so to Bed

Devilish disaster

On the rainy Monday afternoon of 6 April 1668, Samuel Pepys went to a cockfight, which he thought no great sport.

> And thence to the park in a hackney-coach, so would not go into the Tour, but round about the park and to

the House, and there at the door eat and drank; whither came my Lady Kerneagy, of whom Creed tells me more perticularly: how her Lord, finding her and the Duke of York at the King's first coming in too kind, did get it out of her that he did dishonour him; and so he bid her continue to let him, and himself went to the foulest whore he could find, that he might get the pox; and did, and did give his wife it on purpose, that she (and he persuaded and threatened her that she should) might give it the Duke of York; which she did, and he did give it the Duchesse; and since, all her children are thus sickly and infirm – which is the most pernicious and foul piece of revenge that ever I heard of. And he at this day owns it with great glory, and looks upon the Duke of York and the world with great content in the ampleness of his revenge.

This story told Pepys by the Earl of Sandwich's servant John Creed has been disclosed regularly since 1665, by the Comte de Gramont (who was Anthony Hamilton), by Gilbert Burnet (who was Bishop of Salisbury) and by a London doctor I met last week in a pub (who swore it happened in the 1960s to the wife of a cabinet minister).

28

Luckless Lübeck

Vaccine backfires

'My brother was an invalid,' recounted Anthony Trollope, 'and the horrid word, which of all words was, for some years after, the most dreadful to us, had been pronounced. . . . My younger sister Emily, with that false-tongued hope which knows the truth, but will lie lest the heart should faint, had been called delicate, but only delicate, was now ill. Of course she was doomed.'

The unspeakable word today is cancer. In 1834 it was consumption. Trollope's brother Henry was dead by Christmas, Emily two years later at eighteen, four of his children died from it between twelve and thirty-three. His contemporary Dickens named it the disease which 'medicine never cured, wealth never warded off'.

'Captain of all these men of death that came against him to take him away,' wrote John Bunyan about Mr Badman, 'was the Consumption, for it was that that brought him down to the grave.' (Tuberculosis is the most literary of diseases.)

The Captain led most British and Americans into eternal captivity from the end of the eighteenth century to the middle of the next. Napoleon ravaged Europe but tuberculosis filled a quarter of its graves. In the Eastern States it killed 5 in 1000 Americans, 130 in 1000 if they happened to be in gaol (and white, the black rates were worse). Quaker physician Thomas Young confessed consumption 'so fatal as to deter practitioners from attempting a cure'.

Familiar names are carved on the Captain's memorial. Charlotte and Emily Brontë, coughing over each other behind closed windows amid the Yorkshire moors, their two sisters already dead. Robert Louis Stevenson hopelessly seeking health in Samoa, George Orwell turning as desperately to Scotland, D. H. Lawrence to Nice, the *Yellow Book*'s Aubrey Beardsley to Menton. Dr Anton Chekhov at forty-four, Edgar Allan Poe and Franz Kafka at forty. Raphael, Watteau and Modigliani. Paganini, Purcell, Chopin and Mozart. Mimi and Louis Dubedat on stage.

'I know the colour of that blood,' cried Dr John Keats the first time he spat it. 'It is arterial blood, I cannot be deceived in that colour. That drop of blood is my death warrant – I must die.'

Lying fevered and wasting in his little square room by the Spanish Steps in Rome, Keats implored his devoted friend, the painter Joseph Severn, 'You must not look at me in my dying gasp, nor breathe my passing breath.' Few were so worried that consumption might be catching. Its prevalence masked its infectivity. It seemed an affliction as natural as death itself.

The Verona physician Heronymous Frascastorius suspected it was contagious in 1546. In England two hundred years later, Dr Benjamin Martin's *New Theory of Consumption* depicted anamalculae fretting and gnawing in stomach, liver and lungs. Professor Rudolf Virchow of Berlin – whose microscope magnified Sir Morell Mackenzie's bungles with the Crown Prince's larynx – thought tuberculosis invaded the body with deadly bundles of cells, like cancer.

Robert Koch was a Rhineland country doctor, who with Louis Pasteur became to germs what Copernicus and Galileo were to the stars. In 1882 he found the cause of tuberculosis, a slender bacillus which grasped a crimson stain too firmly for decolorization with acids – the 'acid-fast' bacillus. Many physicians retained their clinical ideas as forcefully. Germs remained German fancies, while death rose from the widespread habit of spitting on the floor.

The cause was found, the cure yearned for. In 1890 Koch was cascaded with honours for discovering it – 'tuberculin', a glycerine extract of the bacillus. It was a false claim, the only taint in a career of pure benefaction. The White Plague diminished as the century extended, through better feeding and housing. Dr S. Adolphus Knopf of Philadelphia recognized in 1901, 'To combat consumption successfully requires the combined action of a wise government, well-trained physicians, and an intelligent people.' Applied to diseases now filling the Captain's stealthy boots, the idea could do us a lot of good.

In 1922, Drs Calmette and Guérin vaccinated a child with attenuated cow TB, producing immunity to the human disease. There was not even a painful injection, you swallowed it. Every parent wanted so sure, so safe a way of saving his family. And if tuberculosis could be prevented in individuals, surely it could be eliminated from the world?

In the spring of 1930, some children given Bacille Calmette–Guérin in the German port of Lübeck became ill. One died. It caused no stir. Children were always being ill at that time of year. Then another 14 died. Prophyaxis with BCG stopped. Of 249 children vaccinated between 24 February and 25 April, 73 were dead by autumn. Those dosed in the ten days of mid-March and the end of April suffered nine-tenths of the deaths.

No secret virulence could have surged in the harmless culture of germs, supplied by the Institute Pasteur in Paris. A hundred children vaccinated from the same batch across the Baltic at Riga were fine. The Minister of the Interior had interested himself when the number of dead children reached 52. For a politician to ride a tragedy, he fires criminal charges from the saddle. The hospital, the children's clinic, four laboratory directors were accused of manslaughter.

The police found that the stock of deadly doses and the original germs from Paris had mysteriously been destroyed. Doctors gossiped about a virulent vial of human TB germs from Kiel, which had lost its label in the same Lübeck laboratory. Inquisitive Dr Ludwig Lange found a forgotten ampoule of the vanished vaccine, and grew its bacilli in bacteriologists' nutrative soup. A green tinge developed, unusual with BCG germs. He tried growing the Kiel germs. They produced green, too. He grew germs taken from the victims' corpses. Green as well.

The coincidence suggested that an unknown patient in Kiel had fatally infected 73 children in Lübeck. The murderous muddle could not be proved. The hospital, the clinic, the laboratory directors were cleared after a long trial. The disaster was forgotten. People were anyway distracted that year by Hitler declaring himself ready to capture the soul of Germany.

In 1930, 12 youngsters died among 559 vaccinated with BCG at Ujpest, Hungary, and one from 10 at Santiago. The vaccine is today given medical students and nurses, and advised for susceptible children. The inoffensive, unconsidered vole has scampered to man's aid. The tuberculosis bacillus which kills voles bestows human immunity. It is innocuous to man, and does not need the labour of attenuation in a laboratory.

No longer 'Youth grows pale, and spectre thin, and dies.' For near a century, youth fought the fell Captain on the battlefields of Davos, Montreux, St Moritz, living languorously up mountains in the guaranteed Swiss air. Dr Edward Livingstone Trudeau – who saw a doctor's duty 'to cure sometimes, to relieve often, to comfort always' – founded a native sanatorium in 1882 at Saranac Lake in the Adirondacks. He had developed TB himself, after walking one night the length of New York from Central Park to the Battery in forty-seven minutes for a bet.

The conjunction of character and circumstance in sanatoria was irresistible to Thomas Mann and Dr Somerset Maugham (a casualty), particularly as the fever made the victims sexy. The antibiotic streptomycin overcame tuberculosis in the 1950s. It also knocked the bottom out of the Swiss sanatorium market. They became hotels advertising their deep, airy, sunny balconies. I wonder how many people died on them.

29

The Decline and Fall of Edward Gibbon

Inexpressible embarrassment

Edward Gibbon was fat and foppish. His literary opponents ridiculed both the affliction and the affectation. He also suffered from gout.

He got the idea for *Decline and Fall* in the Capitol ruins at Rome on 15 October 1765, and finished it towards midnight in a summerhouse at Lausanne on 27 June 1787. On 11 November 1793, he wrote from St James's in London to his friend and editor Lord Sheffield in Sussex.

I must at length withdraw the veil before my state of health though the naked truth may alarm you more than a fit of the gout. Have you never observed through my *inexpressibles* a large prominency which, as it was not at all painful and very little troublesome I have strangely neglected for many years? But since my departure from Sheffield Place it has increased (most stupendously), is increasing and ought to be diminished. Yesterday I sent for Farquhar who is allowed to be a very skilful surgeon. After viewing and palpating he desired to call in assistance and has examined it again today with Mr Cline, a surgeon, as he says, of the first eminence. They both pronounce it a hydrocele (a collection of water) which must be let out by the operation of tapping, but from its magnitude and long neglect they think it a most extraordinary case and wish to have another surgeon, Dr Baille present. If the business should go off smoothly I shall be delivered from my burden (it is almost as big as a small child) and walk about in four or five days with a truss. But the medical gentlemen, who never speak quite plain, insinuate to me the possibility of an inflammation, of fever, etc.

It was a disastrous decision.

Hydrocele is a benign and common scrotal condition. The operation performed a few days later produced four quarts of clear fluid, the burden reduced by half. A cruel relief. A fortnight later the lump grew as big as ever, the draining repeated. The fluid returned again, the insinuated inflammation gripped, the operation site was covered with ulcers.

By 9 January 1794, Gibbon ran a high fever. Four days later, the surgeons made a third incision and took six quarts. Next morning he seemed better, the next he suffered sickness and abdominal pain, treated with warm napkins and opium. He rose after a wretched night at 8.30, returned to bed for Mr Farquhar at eleven. The surgeon found his patient collapsed, shook his head and left. Edward Gibbon took some brandy at noon, and threequarters of an hour later was dead.

He was fifty-six. Had he let well alone, he might have lived to the Battle of Waterloo. He could have emulated the treatment of Mr Robert Liston's patient with the wheelbarrow. He suffered the slowly growing hydrocele for thirty-two years, since first consulting the surgeon Mr Hawkins. Had he submitted to eighteenth-century surgery then, much of the world would never have known the grandeur that was Rome, and Gibbon would be remembered as a captain on the rolls of the Hampshire militia.

30

The Sack-'em-Up Men

Disaster for Scottish anatomy

'Heal the sick, cleanse the lepers, raise the dead, cast out devils,' Jesus sent forth his disciples, knowing of course the forthcoming split of medicine into therapeutics, epidemiology, resuscitation and psychiatry.

The Early Christians obeyed with evangelical zeal. They claimed exclusive world rights in healing, prescribing prayer and fasting. The human body was sacred, never to be violated by dissection (the Moslems agreed). Religion thus immobilized medicine for fifteen centuries.

A doctor who has never run his fingers through a body is an astronomer without a telescope. Galen in the 1800s did his best with Barbary apes. The Renaissance anatomist Andreas Versalius founded his career on luckily discovering outside the walls of Louvain a criminal's skeleton hanging in chains, complete with ligaments. When Henry VIII decreed in 1540 that surgeons were a cut above barbers, he awarded them two executed criminals a year for dissection.

From gallows and gibbet came medicine's greatest bene-
factors. Anatomy schools flourished with the hangmen in
the eighteenth century. Windmill Street in Soho had Scotsman William Hunter's famous Theatre of Anatomy, con-
tinuing the tradition two centuries later with London's first
strip show. In 1717 Edinburgh appointed its first professor
of anatomy, aged twenty-two. There was sometimes a wee
fret over students posing as mourners and snatching the
body. One newly executed woman revived during a fight
over hers, and lived on for years as 'Half-hangit Maggie'.

The official Edinburgh University anatomists suffered
competition from able extramural teachers with a robust,
showbiz approach, lecturing in a rivalry which infected
their devoted students. All needed to keep 'the table' ad-
quately furnished. Six taught in Surgeons' Square, by the
Infirmary in High School Yards, with its adjoining plot for
burying unclaimed bodies. This was to the students an
academic convenience as prized as the Bodleian at Oxford.

Snatching a body is easier than catching a salmon.

1. Wait till dark.
2. Post a couple of lookouts against rival
   resurrectionists and excitable relatives.
3. Dig a hole in the loose earth *at the head* of the grave.
   Use a flat, daggerlike spade of *wood*, to avoid noise
   with the stones. Spread canvas sheet for soil,
   keeping grass uncontaminated.
4. Apply two hooks to coffin lid, pull with rope,
   splinter lid (pack hole with sacks to muffle cracking
   noise).
5. Take body *by both ears*, extract.
6. Replace shroud. That would be stealing. A body
   belongs to nobody.
7. Sack up body.
8. Make good, remove tools from site, decamp.

It should take an hour.

The most popular anatomist in Edinburgh was Dr Robert Knox, his rooms a three-storey balconied and porticoed

house at No. 10 Surgeons' Square, jammed between Surgeons' Hall and the Royal Medical Society. In the winter of 1828 he was teaching 504 pupils, threequarters of the whole medical school. He was thirty-seven, claimed descent from John 'Monstrous Regiment of Women' Knox, had German blood, once treated the wounded at Waterloo, was as much part of the Edinburgh scene as Arthur's Seat.

He was dome-headed and side-whiskered, sharp-nosed with a jutting lower lip, chin lost in high collar, festooned with golden watch chains and seals, a diamond cravat ring, little round glasses, one-eyed like Mr Squeers. He was contentious, caustic, cynical, vain, evasive and spiteful. He lectured his students with relish about Robert Liston mistaking a neck aneurism for an abscess, killing a patient in the next-door Infirmary – odd, because they were telling the story six years later set in London, with the fragment in a jar to prove it (see Chapter 1, Triple Knock-Out). Perhaps Liston made a habit of it.

Knox was an enthusiastic raconteur, a gripping lecturer. He needed to repeat each discourse thrice a day to a crammed lecture room of applauding students. He loved anatomy as Romeo Juliet.

Fee for the course was £3 5s, extra for 'subjects' (guaranteed fresh). For his own demonstrations, his pupils' dissections, Knox had a logistical problem. He was paying £800 a year to sportive students and Edinburgh's lurking resurrectionists, which today would have bought his consultant's Rolls-Royce.

On the night of 29 November 1827, two new suppliers brought Dr Knox an old man in a sack and got £7 10s. They had intended taking it to the university's Professor Monro, which would have saved Dr Knox much trouble, the couple being Burke and Hare.

The corpse was an army pensioner who had died in Hare's lodging house at Tanner's Close in slummy West Port beyond Grassmarket, beneath the castle. He owed the landlord £4, and lodger Burke agreed the loss could be justifiably cleared by turning the debtor into a 'shot for the doctor'. They cracked open the coffin, popped the corpse back to bed, and replaced it with a sack of tanner's bark over which the scanty mourners squeezed their tears.

William Burke was short and spry, adept at the jig, nimble-witted and affable. William Hare had a skew face, left eye higher than right, large thick-lipped mouth, hollow cheeks, and laughed a lot. His tumbledown two-storey house was crammed with beds (threepence a night, but you had to share with a couple). Privacy lay in a small back room overlooking a pigsty. Both men had come from Ireland to work on the Union Canal being dug between Edinburgh and Glasgow.

The pair were appalled at the profligacy of letting rot underground something worth £7 10s – particularly as the doctor cordially implied he would be glad to see them with more. Where from? Unfortunately the dead did not hang on every tree. Retailers Burke and Hare, like Marks and Spencer and Saks, Fifth Avenue, decided to create their own products.

A miller in Hare's house was ill of the fever, annoyingly repelling customers. They held a pillow over his face. He was likely to die anyway. He fetched £10. On 11 February 1828, they invited into the room over the pigsty an old beggarwoman called Abigail, filled her with whisky, did it by hand, nailed her in a tea chest and delivered her to Dr Knox, who was delighted with her freshness. The split was set at £4 to Burke, £5 to Hare and £1 to Mrs Hare for ancillary duties. It was she who shortly filled a pair of stray women with whisky. Hare did one, Burke the other.

On 9 April, an eighteen-year-old tart, Mary Patterson, was released from a night in the Canongate watch house. She met Burke in a tavern, he filled her up with rum and bitters, took her home for breakfast (tea, bread, eggs, Finnan haddies), poured her a bottle of whisky, she passed out, got done before lunch, was delivered in the afternoon, made £8 (prices were seasonal, less in summer).

Mary Patterson died with tuppence-ha'penny irremovably tight in her hand (cadaveric spasm, occurs before rigor mortis). As the pair had crossed High School Yards with the sack, the boys all jeered they were carrying a corpse. This voluptuous conscript to their instructors provided a nasty turn for several students and Knox's assistant Mr Fergusson (later Sir William Fergusson, Bart., Serjeant-Surgeon to Queen Victoria), who had known her professionally in Canongate. One Velazquez of the scalpel sketched Mary as a defunct Rokeby Venus. Burke cut off her sandy hair. She would have been dissected to bits within four hours of death, but Dr Knox wanted to save her for his lecture on female musculature and kept her in a barrel of whisky three months.

Burke was otherwise a cobbler. An old cinder gatherer called Effie brought him some scraps of leather, was stupefied with whisky, made £10. Early one morning, Burke relieved two policemen of a drunk woman being dragged to West Port watch house, said he knew her lodgings, took her home, got £10 for her.

June came, cleanly breezes blowing from the Forth, chimneys reeking sparsely into the pale blue sky, castle high on its mound as threatening as a thundercloud. An Irishwoman with her twelve-year-old grandson arrived from Gasgow searching for friends, was kindly directed by Burke, invited home, filled with whisky, done. The child was a damnable difficulty. They could take him out and lose him, but he might return with a policeman. Next day he was asking tearfully after grandma, Burke broke his back, they had to use a herring barrel for the pair of them. In the Mealmarket, Hare's horse collapsed between the shafts of his cart, a crowd gathered, they urgently sent to Dr Knox for a porter with a handcart. They got £16 for the pair, the horse went to the knacker's.

On the anniversary of the Battle of Bannockburn, Mrs Hare urged Burke to turn his live-in love Helen McDougall into stock-in-trade, but he took her on holiday to Falkirk instead. Hare meanwhile made £8 on his own account, causing a quarrel which moved Burke to a basement down the lane, sleeping on straw. Like discordant Gilbert and

Sullivan, their prosperity depended on an irksome partnership. They did for Helen's distant cousin Ann (Burke fastidiously had Hare perform the stifling). Dr Knox thought the pair justified a trunk for further supplies (see Chapter 26, Doctor Death).

Next, their charwoman Mrs Hostler (£8), ninepence-ha'-penny gripped in her dead hand. Then Mrs Haldane and her daughter Peggy (tarts). Then eighteen-year-old Daft Jamie, imbecile, well known to Edinburgh and his dissectors (Knox ordered the head removed first). Jamie had put up a fight, bitten Burke, Knox treated him. Finally Mrs Madge Docherty on All Saints Eve. Two lodgers grassed. The police found her in a tea chest in the cellar at No. 10 Surgeons' Square. Early on the Sunday morning of 2 November, Burke and Hare were arrested. Edinburgh erupted. The *Evening Courant* sold an extra 8000 copies an issue.

The trial started at ten in the morning of Christmas Eve. The quality of bench and bar was there, delighting in pawky, rarefied legal quibble. It continued non-stop until 9.30 on Christmas Day, when the jury found Burke guilty. The judge had ordered the windows kept open, the lawyers wrapping their heads against freezing draughts in gowns and coloured handkerchiefs. His only expressed doubts were whether Burke's body should be exhibited in chains or his skeleton preserved as a minatory memento. Hare had spared himself a dreadful night by turning King's evidence.

Burke was hanged in the Lawnmarket at 8.15 on the depressingly wet morning of Wednesday, 18 January 1823, before 25,000 people, including Sir Walter Scott. A view from a window cost 5s to £1. The hangman's entourage fought for fragments of the rope. Burke was taken for dissection to Professor Monro, who next day lectured on his brain (unusually soft). On Friday the public were admitted, 30,000 all day past the black marble slab. His remaining bits were pickled in barrels for future reference. I encountered his scrotum at a delightful dinner of the Royal College of Surgeons of Edinburgh.

As the drop fell the cry rose, 'Hang Knox!' The mob burned his effigy, stormed his house, broke his windows. He was smuggled away cloaked, armed with sword, pistols and skean-dhu, guarded by police. Knox was baffled at the populace implicating him with sixteen murders. A gentleman engrossed in the intellectual intricacies of the human frame frets not over the origin of the anonymous example before him – no more than he would concern himself whether the fine pheasant bought from a villager for his dinner might be poached. Knox was vindicated by a committee of Scottish noblemen and gentry, all appointed by himself. The students he faced began to dwindle, the animosities to rise. In ten years he was out of Surgeons' Square, in fifteen out of work.

Like Robert Liston, Knox turned his back on his unforgiving countrymen for London. He wrote about whales and did obstetrics in Hackney, where he died of apoplexy aged seventy-one. Hare was last seen wandering two miles south of Carlisle across the English border, on Sunday morning 8 February 1829. Burke lives in the eternal glory of the *Oxford English Dictionary* – 'To kill secretly by suffocation or strangulation . . . "hush up", suppress quietly.'

Burke and Hare bestowed Lord Warburton's Anatomy Act of 1832. Matters are better regulated now. If you wish to leave yourself for medical students, fill in form AA1 (obtainable from Her Majesty's Inspector of Anatomy, issued with full instructions). They send their own hearse and coffin, and have to pay for your eventual fragmented funeral.

31

A Lousy Trick

Itching for revenge

A frightful thing happened at Cambridge in 1522. His Majesty's judge, gorgeously robed, convened with lawyers in wigs and gowns, brilliantly uniformed sheriffs, the university vice-chancellor in academicals, the chaplain in canonicals, the mayor in full municipal fig, the trumpeters, criers and pikemen. They were trying the wretches delivered clanking from the county jails, flogging, branding and hanging them, that they might reform their wicked ways. The prisoners exacted terrible retribution. All were jumping with lice, which carry typhus fever (there was a lot of it about in the sixteenth century). 'Gaol fever' was an accepted part of your punishment, like the bread and water. The lice jumped from bar to bench, infected the judicial pageant and perfectly respectable people throughout the town. The 'Black Assizes' was repeated at Oxford in 1577, killing 510 people, and at Exeter in 1589, decimating Devon.

You are unlikely to catch typhus in the splendidly appointed gaols of the West, but it is another reason for behaving yourself in the USSR.

32

The Black Death

A clerical disaster

Shortly before the feast of St John the Baptist in 1348, two ships from Bristol berthed at Melcombe in Dorset. One of the sailors had brought from Gascony 'the seeds of the terrible pestilence'. Melcombe enjoys remembrance as the first town in England ravaged by the Black Death.

Pasteurella pestis is a delicate round germ with a clear centre, like a Polo mint. It is transmitted by rat fleas, producing bubonic plague with 'buboes' of swollen lymph glands in the groins. The Black Death was its pneumonic form, a lethal infection causing gangrene of the lungs passed round as easily as flu and colds.

The dead were black from haemorrhages into their skin. Corpses putrefied in houses and the streets, fearfully untouched. Pits were hastily dug and as rapidly filled – 'the testator and his heirs and executors were hurled from the same cart into the same hole together'. There was no more protection than from the lightning. Families burned juniper for fumigation, the sick tried blood-letting or swallowing vinegar as advised by the 'plague tracts'. The physicians dressed up like modern surgeons, gloves, gown, mask with sponge soaked in cloves and cinnamon. Coast dwellers put to sea, and found the pestilence their cargo. Others fled their villages, forsaking friends, parents, children, efficiently spreading the infection.

The people had no doctors. They called in the clergy to save their lives by divine intercession, or failing that their souls by confession. Over the winter of 1348, a hundred Dorset clergymen died. The vicars of Shaftesbury and Wareham were replaced four times between December and May. In neighbouring Somerset, the usual 9 new clergymen a month increased in December to 32, in January to 47, February to 43, March to 36. Forty-eight per cent of the clergy died in the West Country diocese of Bath and Wells. The parishioners marvelled at the man of God perishing just like his miserable sinners.

In January 1349, their Bishop wrote,

> The contageous pestilence of the present day, which is spreading far and wide, has left many parish churches and other livings in our diocese without parson or priest to care for their parishioners. Since no priests can be found who are willing, whether out of zeal and devotion or in exchange for a stipend, to take on the pastoral care of these aforesaid places, nor to visit the sick and administer to them the Sacraments of the Church (perhaps for fear of infection and contagion), we understand that many people are dying without the Sacrament of Penance.

He announced a sensational emergency relaxation of canonical rules, permitting dying confession to another layman, 'even to a woman'. The Bishop's exhortation dutifully to succour the sick was enfeebled by his passing the plague shut away in his house in the inaccessible village of Wiveliscombe.

Of an English population of four million, 33 per cent died in the Black Death. Of parish priests, 45 per cent. Of the pious 17,500 secluded in monasteries and nunneries, 51 per cent from infection penetrating the susceptible cloisters.

Like the British Army in World War One, the Church lost its best and keenest young officers. Like Britain afterwards, it felt their lack. The sufferings of the Black Death left a land stirring with discontent and doubt, and left manor and parsonage ineffective to answer them.

It seems dreadfully unfair, or at least short-sighted, of God.

'How do you explain the scourges that afflict mankind?' a gentle old lady asked an Abbé in *The Revolt of the Angels*. 'Why are there plagues, famines, floods and earthquakes?'

'It is surely necessary that God should sometimes remind us of his existence,' the Abbé replied with a heavenly smile.

33

Everyday Disaster

A risk ready reckoner

Driving a car for 4000 miles = the same risk as smoking 100 cigarettes = 2 hours' rock climbing = 1 year working in the chemical industry. The risk of riding a motorbike for 350 hours = drinking 40 bottles of wine = eating 80 jars of peanut butter. Magically removing all other causes of death, a steelworker doing 2000 hours a year would live to be 6000, a man driving a car 10 hours a week would die aged 3500, riding a motorbike aged only 300. Anyone smoking 40 cigarettes a day would just make 100. Professor Trevor Kletz of Loughborough University, England, says so.

For disaster, there's no place like home. Sixteen hours a day at home for 2 years = those 350 hours on the motorbike. Most accidents happen at home. Over 500 British children under five are killed there every year – choking on playthings, suffocating in plastic bags, scalding themselves in the kitchen, falling downstairs and into the fire, poisoning themselves with grown-ups' pretty drug capsules. The tragedy of these tragedies is that with parental foresight and common sense most are preventable.

Hospitals are worse. The public has known for centuries what dangerous places they were. Now University Hospital, Boston, has proved it. Of 815 patients there during 1980 290 were suffering from the effects of their treatment (iatrogenesis = Greek for 'caused by physicians'), 76 seriously so, and 15 were shortly killed by it. Modern doctors are prodigal with drugs and tests. This is partly from admir-

able conscientiousness, partly from terror of being sued for
negligence, partly because in many countries they come
completely free (except for their taxpayers). But mostly
because these risky remedies and hazardous investigations
allow patients to scrape through a succession of formerly
fatal illnesses.

Three other disasters of modern living –

A London girl aged fifteen used her teeth to unscrew the
metal cap on a plastic bottle of orange juice. It had fer-
mented during two months outside a refrigerator, and blew
up. She arrived in hospital pouring blood from her mouth.
The surgeons could see down her throat the bared, pulsating left carotid artery – had this been severed, death from
exsanguination or from suffocation in her own blood would
have been an academic point. She recovered, but her tonsils
had been avulsed. It was no compensation for the poor girl
to be the only case in surgical history of tonsillectomy
performed by explosive.

The seventeen-year-old daughter of a Bristol (England)
video-games engineer played with them two hours a day
in his workshop. Space Invader, Asteroids, Space Fury,
Defender, Lunar Rescue, no trouble. With Dark Warrior,
she collapsed. Distraught father imagined her electrocuted,
rushed her to hospital. She was sensitive to the multicol-
oured flashing lights and had a fit, the first case of Dark
Warrior epilepsy. A young Roumanian had previously suffered Astro Fighter epilepsy. You can also get a sprained
wrist from them.

The 1960s had a mini-disaster. The second female curse
(cystitis) spread with short skirts and the substitution of
tights for stockings and suspenders. The close-fitting nylon
invited infection by retaining moisture and heat while excluding air. Tights were such a bother to get down, the risk
increased as the ladies peed so much less frequently.

And watch out in the woods. The Death Cap toadstool
(*Amanita phalloides*) causes 90 per cent of deaths from fungus

poisoning. You see it among the trees all summer, dirty white satiny cap, white gills, white ring dangling from stem and ragged sheath rising from foot. It is disastrously confused with an edible mushroom. The antidote is known only to Dr Pierre Bastien in Remiremont, a small town in the Vosges, who ate them sautéd on television to prove it. The False Death Cap (*Amanita citrina*) is similar, but smells of raw potato. It may be eaten with impunity. It is best not to try.

Every year, bees and wasps kill one in ten million among the population of Britain, Western Europe and the United States. This is more than killed by atomic energy, but causes less fuss.

34

Love Locked In

Dubious disaster

The film *What's Up Nurse?* had an amorous couple on British Rail who got jammed, in the loo. Note comma.

Amid flashing blue lights, shrieking sirens and scarlet blankets, they sped for surgical disentanglement. (It was a doctor up nurse, dreadfully *infra dig* in casualty.) This operation is as fictional as the penis transplant in *Percy*, the movie which did better business in its native Britain than *The Sound of Music*.

Penis captivus was well known in the Middle Ages. It was God's punishment for copulating among the owls and bats in night-shrouded churches and churchyards. Release was effected at cockcrow, by prayers and buckets of cold water.

The first case recorded by a doctor was in 1729, the next in 1923 at Warsaw, in the park. The couple were so ashamed when it got in the papers, they shot themselves.

The Sexual Life of Our (1908) *Time* describes another in Bremen docks. 'A great crowd assembled, from the midst of which the unfortunate couple were removed in a closed carriage, and taken to the hospital, and not until chloroform had been administered to the girl did the spasm pass off and free the man.' For another case, two years later, they had to crack ice as well.

Alfresco furtive fornication was blamed. Nervous contraction of powerful muscles round the vagina trapped the erect penis, like a sailing ship in a bottle. Such fearsome spasm was powerfully augmented by the rapid gathering of a crowd not sympathetically inclined to the girl's blushes.

It was not always a vicious vice. It could clamp in the marriage bed. One new wife in the 1860s suffered a springtime of treatment 'which involved the application of a probe, speculum, compressive sponge, glycerine tampons, etc. . . . This young and chronically neurotic woman grew every week more agitated and excitable so that she eventually responded to the smallest aggravation with compulsive crying fits.'

Her husband bravely tried a cure through a natural application, and escaped with bruises.

The captive penis has not arisen this century. Cases of foreskin hooked on an intrauterine device like a rising trout do not count. Penis captivus is perhaps as much a mythical Victorian disease as clergyman's sore throat or scriveners' palsy. Should it strike on the back seat of your Fiesta, it is best to blow down each others' nostrils. It seems to work with horses.

35

Suffer the Little Children
If politically advantageous

In 1971 a Tory Minister of Education abolished the free milk which schoolchildren had been imbibing each noon since the Battle of Britain, or possibly Agincourt.

Every country has its explosive political conjunctions. In Germany, Nazi and past. In France, minister and mistress. In Italy, mayor and Mafia. In America, President and his family.

In Britain, it is children and milk.

Labour was outraged, unbelieving, furious. It saddled the Tories with transmuting the burgeoning generation into a sickly pack of wizened midgets. The Tories thought the money should be spent on something useful, like books.

Merthyr Tydfil in the green valleys of South Wales had the tenderest regard for little children, or one of the heftiest Labour parliamentary majorities in the country. Putting humanity before mortification, its town council voted to defy the Queen's writ and went on delivering the milk of human kindness. Martyrdom lasted a month, until the borough treasurer refused to sign cheques for the dairy.

Merthyr Tydfil council eyed aghast its bright-eyed, lilting-voiced youngsters, who would perish without milk as surely as premature infants in their incubators. The effect on Welsh rugby football was unthinkable. Like Thomas Gray, they tremblingly let 'regardless of their doom, The little victims play'. The doom was documented seven years later by the Medical Research Council in Cardiff.

The doctors followed 581 Welsh eight-year-olds, all with 3 or more brothers and sisters, 571 of them from 'working-class' families, 134 with fathers on the dole, and 46 from the socially infamous single-parent families.

Half had milk every schoolday, half not. The milk-drinking boys became averagely 0·11 centimetres shorter and 0·21 kilograms fatter, the girls 0·45 centimetres taller and 0·05 kilograms fatter – figures which 'do not achieve statistical significance. . . . The reintroduction of free school milk for seven- to eleven-year-old children is unlikely to have any appreciable effect on the physical development of the children.'

In 1974 mercy returned to British politics with another Labour government. Its Minister of Education, Mrs Shirley Williams, restored free school milk despite the Minister of Health imploring her not to. The milk was offered cut-price by the European Economic Community, which has the compassion towards little ones of the Merthyr Tydfil town council, and an enormous milk surplus.

The fatter the milk the fatter the EEC subsidy, which made the Coronary Prevention Group furious. *Over*nutrition is now our children's problem, and the poor little things will all drop dead from heart attacks at thirty. The British genius for compromise is being directed towards skimmed milk.

Politically you cannot tell milk from lead. Whether lead turns your children into shambling morons depends on your vote. The humanitarian Labour party is committed headlong to expunging lead from petrol. The Tories are more wary of the scientists' conflicting reports. Of 166 children living near a London leadworks, those with low lead-levels were found to be more scholastically accomplished, *but* they were sixteen months older than the high-lead-level ones. Besides, many Tory voters have oil shares in their portfolios. Pornography has a similar effect on the brain to lead, seen from different political poles. Tobacco emits Calverley's sublime fragrance for its workers' union, and nuclear annihilation seems not nearly so bad if you are a right-winger.

Politicians' habitual irrational response to proven facts is frightening, but the papers would be disastrously dull without it.

Stopping the milk did not retard the career of the Tory
minister, who was Mrs Thatcher.

36

Kinky Kinks

Corset disaster

Your nuciform sac is full of decaying matter –
undigested food and waste products – rank ptomaines.
Now you take my advice, Ridgeon. Let me cut it out
for you. You'll be another man afterwards.

Mr Cutler Walpole on 20 November 1906, on the stage of
the Court Theatre, London. The play was Shaw's *Doctor's
Dilemma*.

Across the Thames, Sir William Arbuthnot Lane, Bart.,
starred in the theatre of Guy's Hospital.

Many are obsessed with their bowels. Sir William was
obsessed with the bowels of the earth. The colon – the last
lap of the guts – he saw coiled in the abdomen like a snake
in the grass. A static, solid, seething sac of putrefying
provisions, its poisons absorbed by the bloodstream to ruin
physical and psychological health. Constipation! Chronic
intestinal stasis! Auto-intoxication! he diagnosed frenziedly. He described an everyday case.

> The sensation imparted to the hand of the observer by
> that of the toxic patient is unmistakable. It is cold and
> clammy, and moist on its palmar surface. The ears are
> also bluish and feel cold, as also does the nose. . . The
> loss of fat in the face and neck produces an appearance
> of age, distress and disappointment which is most
> pathetic, particularly in the young subject. . . . The
> individual is also unable to lead an active physical life
> because of poor muscular development.

He also had 'a nasty graveyard odour'.

Sir William Lane reads much like Dr William Acton (see Chapter 12, Disastrous Habits). If the patients masturbated as well, God knows what they looked like.

The colon was perpetually loaded, how could he fire it of faeces? He tried a pint of cream a day, and so much liquid paraffin that a match applied to the fundament would have illuminated the drawing room. He had men wear body belts, ladies change their corsets – 'The English corset is disastrous. . . . The straight-busked French corset is much less harmful.'

Then he discovered Lane's kink, and surgically short-circuited it. Fair enough. Had you taken your symptoms to the man next door in Cavendish Square, he would as eagerly have anchored your floating kidneys, buoyed up your sinking stomach or divided your invisible adhesions. Doctors are slaves to fashion like dress designers.

In the 1900s, Lane met Elie Metchnikoff, Russian Nobel Prize winner. He had written a book proving the entire one and a half yards of colon a useless, vestigial structure, like the appendix. It was the meeting of pope and crusader. Lane afterwards removed his patients' colons as nonchalantly as shaking their clammy hands. A boy misdirected from a throat surgeon had his colon removed instead of his tonsils. A man who tried cutting his throat nearly had his wife's colon removed, to better her temper and reduce domestic suicidal pressure.

Sir William had his critics. 'Encouraged by us doctors,' declared another medical knight just before World War One, 'hundreds and thousands of human beings have grafted into themselves the idea that they were born into the world for the main purpose of getting a daily evacuation of their bowels, for should they fail in this they will be poisoned by the absorption of the noxious products that are, they suppose, forming in this their kitchen garden.'

The garden grew Sir William £10,000 a year.

Lane died during World War Two aged eighty-six, outliving his operation by thirty years. He was not Cutler

Walpole of the fictional nuciform sac. Shaw confessed his original 'a laryngeal specialist who extirpated uvulas'. Which is equally effective treatment for constipation, a meaningless term depending wholly on personal standards, like insomnia and pornography.

37

The Dying Art
Hamfisted hangmen

A dwindling posse of nations arms itself with judicial killing, but the scaffold is not yet a piece of incomprehensible furniture. The House of Commons was still debating it in 1982. Enthusiasts and abhorrers should be clear what they argue about. What could put it plainer than Sir Sydney Smith's *Forensic Medicine*?

The execution is carried out as follows:
The prisoner is placed on a platform above trap doors which open downwards when a bolt is drawn. A rope is looped round the neck with the knot under the angle of the jaw and with a sufficient length of rope to allow a drop of five to seven feet according to the weight of the person.
On pulling the bolt the condemned individual drops to the length of the rope; the sudden stoppage of the moving body associated with the position of the knot causes the head to be jerked violently, dislocating or fracturing the cervical column and rupturing the cord. The dislocation often takes place between the second and third cervical vertebrae. Death is instantaneous, although the heart may continue to beat for several minutes. This method of execution is very expeditious and cleanly.
The postmortem appearances are of no consequence.

From Sir Sydney, hanging seems as efficient as tooth-drawing and sounds less painful.

Even inhumanity is bedevilled by human error. Mr Berry in the 1890s, a breezy Yorkshireman whose hobby was otter hunting, was the Escoffier, the Pavlova, the Lord Lister of hanging. He brought style and science to the scaffold. He invented a formula to calculate the drop (aiming at a striking force of twenty-four hundredweight). He assessed each victim's neck tissues with the assiduousness of a throat surgeon.

Even Homer sometimes nods. So did this Homeric hangman. He failed with Mr John Lee, a joyous bungle for the subject tempered by Mr Berry's immediately trying to rectify his error by stringing him up again twice in succession. On 30 November 1895, Mr Robert Goodale's head jerked off at Norwich Castle, but the coroner excused Mr Berry for only a slip in his arithmetic. He almost pulled another one off in Liverpool on 20 August 1891, Mr John Conway's, but that was the fault of heeding the prison doctor, who was pushing his own pamphlet *Judicial Hanging*.

Less academic hangmen of the nineteenth century faced messier results. The disappearance through the trap in Durham of Mr Matthew Atkinson, a local miner, was followed by a dull thud below and a snapped rope above. He had nothing worse than a dislocated jaw, and it took twenty-four minutes before they could rig everything up and hang him again.

Mr John Coffey suffered the same mishap, retrieved from the pit with blood spurting from his ears. The rope annoyingly broke again, but someone neatly caught him before he hit bottom. The third time they strangled him and it took twelve minutes, one hour and one minute less than needed for Mr Antonio Sprecage in Canada.

With Mr Patrick Harnet, 'a heavy gurgling sound was heard, and soon the blood in torrents commenced pouring on the stone floor below'. Hangman Marwood – with whom Mr Berry enjoyed the relationship of brilliant houseman to senior surgeon – dropped Mr Brownless too far and embedded a one-and-a-half inch rope in his neck, blood every-where. (This also occurred in Durham, a city to be avoided for murder.) Mr Berry himself shuddered at anything thicker than threequarters of an inch, comprising five strands of silky Italian hemp, four strands for women.

The executioner of four men in a British colony in 1927 was in a hurry to go and hang some more, so he did them in pairs. The surgeon discovered one groaning and gasping after his hasty departure. All four bodies were suspended for another fifteen minutes, just to make sure.

It was murmured that the last woman hanged in Britain needed a burly warder to score success with a rugby foot-ball tackle.

Expert hands have now lost their art with disuse, like fan-painters. The natural extinction of the professional hangman is surely the best argument for his abolition. What is worth doing at all is worth doing well.

Energetic, imaginative American scientific ingenuity, which gave the world anaesthesia, provided also electro-cution. The advantages were glaring – no danger of the head coming off, it would be nice for the subject to sit down, the chance of a snapped rope was greater than a blown fuse. Mr William Kemmler blazed the trail on 6 August 1890 at Auburn, NY. Only spoilsports suggest that the legal 2000 volts stuns, death coming from the legal postmortem immediately afterwards.

The modern guillotine was equally convenient. You stepped to a board like a pier-mirror, in the fresh air (and before an admiring audience until recently), were securely strapped, smoothly tipped to the horizontal, secured with a stout wooden collar, *et voilà*!

This great labour-saving device was invented by Dr Joseph-Ignace Guillotin on 10 October 1789. He was anx-ious that *égalité* should enjoy its logical conclusion. Like other social events in Europe, public executions were pla-gued by snobbery. Nobles were decapitated, the rabble hanged. The aristocrats took beheading seriously. It would never do to lose their dignity as well. The second Queen whom King Henry VIII sent to the block spent the night before rehearsing.

The prototype guillotine was painstakingly tested with live sheep and dead people, and at 3.30 p.m. on 25 April 1792 M. Nicholas-Jacques Pelletier incited its maiden drop in the Place de Grève. The machine quickly appeared as toys, souvenirs, earrings. It caught public fancy like the yo-yo.

Unlike hanging and electrocution, where the heart trips on merrily for minutes, you were blatantly dead when bundled, in two pieces, into the long wicker box like a music-hall artiste's wardrobe skip.

Or were you?

'An old *surveillant* at St Jean,' wrote Somerset Maugham, 'tells a story of how a doctor had arranged with a man who was to be guillotined to blink three times if he could after his head was cut off, and says he saw him blink twice.'

Dr Frederick Gaertner recounted another disastrous defiance. 'Immediately after the head was severed and dropped in the basket, I took charge of it. The facial expression was that of great agony, for several minutes after decapitation. He would open his eyes, also his mouth, in the process of gaping, as if he wanted to speak to me, and I am positive he could see me for several seconds after the head was severed from the body. There is no doubt that the brain was still active.'

Dr Velpeau in 1864 invited his professional brother Dr de la Pommerais, whom he was going to watch being guillotined in the morning, to blink his right eye three times afterwards in response to his shouted name, but he could manage only once. The head of twenty-four-year-old Charlotte Corday, who four days before murdered Dr Jean-Paul Marat in his bath, blushed indignantly when displayed to the mob. A medical student stuck a scalpel into a newly detached head and produced a grimace. A head tossed into a sack with another bit it. Some corpses ran round for ten minutes like headless chickens.

On 13 November 1879, three doctors were driven by

these tales to experiment on twenty-three-year-old M. Théotime Prunier, shouting in his detached face, sticking in pins, applying ammonia under his nose, silver nitrate and candle flames to his eyeballs. Only response, 'The face bore a look of astonishment.'

Gassing is less accident prone, but miserably unspectacular. The guillotine while it remained on offer was probably the preferable enforcement of a premature end. There was always the outside chance you could spit in your executioner's eye.

38

Clubland Doctor

Disastrous negligence (60 per cent)

Sir Samuel Garth, coming to the Kit Kat club one night, declared he must soon be gone, having many patients to attend; but some good wine being produced he forgot them. Sir Richard Steele was of the party, and reminded him of the visits he had to pay, when Garth immediately pulled out his list, which amounted to fifteen, and said: 'It's no great matter whether I see them tonight or not, for nine of them have such bad constitutions that all the physicians in the world can't save them, and the other six have such good constitutions that all the physicians in the world can't kill them.'

John Timbs (1801–75)

39

Design for Living
Bricks and mortality

'It may seem a strange principle to enunciate as the very first requirement in a Hospital' – Florence Nightingale had a nose for the elusive obvious – 'that it should do the sick no harm.'

She meant architecturally, not clinically.

There was an awesome row in 1856. The Army was building a hospital in Hampshire, to look as impressive upon Southampton Water as the Scutari Selinie Quicklaci upon the Bosphorus. Miss Nightingale damned it from water closet to weathercock.

A Royal Commission tentatively asked if she had devoted attention to hospital design. 'Yes,' Miss Nightingale told them crisply, 'for thirteen years I have visited all the hospitals in London, Dublin and Edinburgh, many county hospitals, some of the naval and military hospitals in England, all the hospitals in Paris and the Institution of Protestant Deaconesses at Kaiserswerth on the Rhine, the hospitals at Berlin and many others in Germany, at Lyons, Rome, Alexandra, Constantinople, Brussels, also the war hospitals of the French and the Sardinians.'

Miss Nightingale knew the best saucepans for the kitchen, the best books for the library, the best colour for the walls (pale pink). And she had written *A Treatise on Sinks*.

The new Army hospital was a brick block pierced by corridors as long as rifle shots. Miss Nightingale wanted a row of pavilions, that the ward air might not mix and contaminate. Like Semmelweis, she countered the activities of germs long before they clinically existed. Her pavilioned shrine of St Thomas's Hospital still edifies Members of Parliament taking tea across the Thames on their terrace.

The Victorian Secretary at War rebuffed her. He could hardly demolish the half-built walls, and at a cost of £70,000. Miss Nightingale spent the weekend with Prime Minister Lord Palmerston. He decided he would rather pay to throw it brick by brick into Southampton Water.

Nobody dared build a hospital in the British Empire without consulting Florence Nightingale. She had never been shipped somewheres east of Suez, but she knew where to look it up. If she ineffectively raged at the Viceroy to open Indian hospital windows in the burning sun and dissipate the precious cool of night, she did it lying in bed all day in Mayfair.

The modern sick are more likely to be harmed by the hospital tumbling about their ears, the newer the building the riskier. The British Department of Health has a £30 million a year bill for hospital defects. The General Hospital at Bangor in Wales needed urgent redesign when someone noticed the pathology department drains went through the kitchen. At the new University Hospital in Cardiff, the roof tiles were flaking like dandruff. The newer Monyhull Geriatric Unit in Birmingham cost £360,000 to build then £88,000 to put right. Other hospitals needed intensive care for incipient collapse at Walsall, Basingstoke, Rhyl, North Ayrshire and Glasgow. The nationwide epidemic struck the world-famous Great Ormond Street Hospital for Children in London. Its new cardiac unit (£7½ million) was evacuated within a year when found to incorporate a DIY earthquake.

Biggest constructional disaster was St George's Hospital at Hyde Park Corner, perfect site for a luxury hotel, views into Buckingham Palace. The Tory Government in 1982 sold it back to the Duke of Westminster for the £23,700 they paid in 1906. It was in the contract. The Labour spokeswoman described the deal as 'extraordinary'. This was the best left-wing British understatement since Clement Attlee always used no words when one would do.

40

Terror in the Tucker
Australian disaster

The equivalent for Australian palates of Thanksgiving turkey, the roast beef of Old England, *saltimbocca alla Romana*, Pekin duck, Beluga caviar, *perdreau en crépine Brillat-Savarin* – possibly of all six combined – is the meat pie.

This is a small tank brimming with gravy the consistency of engine oil, the colour of ashes, and the taste of sheep meat boiled relentlessly and suspectedly whole. The filling has been compared in appearance to 'what little babies do in their nappies'. On biting the casing resembling soggy cardboard, the gravy escapes like superheated steam. To avoid a change of clothing, the pie must be sucked rather than chewed, in the position of bowing reverentially to the Queen.

Such unexpected liquidity is insignificant to the thirsty inhabitants of a land two-thirds desert. They soak the tepid pie in tomato sauce. Some Australians emblazon all their food with tomato sauce – steak, eggs, French fries, oysters, asparagus, *pâté de foie gras*. One incredulous gourmet sampling Australia murmured, 'Your kids take tomato sauce sandwiches to school, and even have been known to put it on their ice cream.'

Australians are addicted to sauce with the reckless indifference of Scotsmen to the variety of whisky cascaded on their haggis. (No Scot has ever tasted haggis. They drink so much whisky first, they would as zestfully be eating boiled knitting.) In 1964, the poisoned chalice was Worcestershire sauce.

A twenty-eight-year-old housewife appeared in Brisbane Hospital with a stone in each kidney. Rigorous investigation on the couch, in the X-ray department, by the biochemistry laboratory, found no cause. Did she swallow popular painkillers? asked the baffled doctors. These can create kidney stones. Overdose herself with vitamin D, in cranky health foods? Drink excessive milk? No? Well, was there *anything* unusual about her diet? Nothing at all, she replied. Unless you count Worcestershire sauce. She had a craving for it. She got through a bottle a day, but more when she was pregnant.

Worcestershire sauce! exclaimed the doctors. Full of acetic acid, which damages the kidney. Plus garlic, black pepper, ginger, allspice, mace, cinnamon, ingredients all containing volatile oils and equally nephrotoxic.

She kicked the habit, the stones grew no bigger. An earlier case then emerged, back in 1956, a bottle-a-day man.

Twelve months later, a twenty-eight-year-old painter appeared at the same hospital. He was a Scots immigrant, so well integrated in his new country he drank six pints of Foster's a day. He never touched milk.

He had two stones in his right kidney, seemingly without cause. Worcestershire sauce? asked the doctors. He was hooked on it. He swamped all his meals with it. His was an addiction tough to break. Like the wayward alcoholic anonymous, the first, quick dash from the bottle was the disastrous one. They dried him out saucewise and the stones stayed static.

I am a Worcestershire sauce buff. A bloody mary, a Welsh rarebit, an Irish stew, are as unmemorable without it as a passionless kiss. After reading these cases I gloomily struggled to renounce it, like cholesterol – a doctor, in the spirit of William Pitt's England, must save himself by his exertions and his patients by his example.

This was *Australian* Worcestershire sauce. The distinction was made with dignified pique in the London *Times* by Mr Lea, who with Mr Perrins makes The Original and Genuine Worcestershire Sauce in Worcester (rhymes with Bertie Wooster), England. Each crimson label carries a brace of grouse, a hare, and their printed signature to discourage imitations, like the Bank of England's notes. The sauce contains shallots, tamarinds and anchovies. It is made from the original recipe of a nobleman, perhaps the incandescent Sir Francis Dashwood of the Hell Fire Club.

No English nobleman would concoct anything remotely damaging to the kidney, an organ cherished by our aristocracy. How many armadas of champagne, port, claret and burgundy have seeped through them since the Battle of Hastings! A peer in his London club – it still had gout stools, to tuck in your chair and raise exquisitely painful toes to the easeful horizontal – so lingered in the bar that the ancient waiter respectfully reminded him of a grill long ordered. 'My Lord, your kidneys are spoiling.' 'My God!' His lordship clasped his loins. 'Is it beginning to show?'

I continue to sprinkle lavishly the English sauce so complimentary to English cooking, which is often inedible if you can taste it.

41

Cleaner Living

Nature adores a vacuum

The loves of senior citizens and venerable monarchs usually provoke ridicule and pity, sometimes admiration and envy, always curiosity.

Every schoolboy sniggers over King David stricken in years, the fair young virgin Abishag lying in his bosom, 'but the king knew her not' – which did not mean they were unacquainted.

King Solomon after his Queen of Sheba phase 'loved many strange women'.

A bare-footed beggar maid affected King Cophetua like a vodka advertisement. In robe and crown the king stept down and sware a royal oath: 'This beggar maid shall be my queen!' Tennyson heard all about it.

King Charles II at forty sired the Duke of St Albans with the help of pretty, witty Nell Gwyn, aged twenty.

Dr Bartolo's eagerness to marry his ward Rosina was thwarted by his nimble-witted barber (baritone). The Lord Chancellor's enthusiasm to marry his ward in Chancery Phyllis was frustrated by the seventeen-year-old mother of the twenty-four-year-old man she *really* wanted to wed, who revealed herself as the Chancellor's wife, turned into a fairy. Opera made sex more complicated than Freud.

Many ageing men fall desperately in love with their vacuum cleaners. Particularly the Hoover 'Dustette' model. These are mistresses more dangerous than Carmen in torrid Seville.

A London man was changing the plug of his 'Dustette' in the nude, while his wife was out shopping, when it inexplicably turned itself on. A railwayman was mysteriously caught in one which happened to be lying about buzzing in his signal box. Another man was hoovering a friend's stairs in a dressing gown, when the suction got him. Another in Denver, Colorado, was vacuuming his car in the back yard, dressed only in his underpants. The cleaner clogged, he sat on the back steps to free it, the motor started unexpectedly and drew him in, as a straw in the wind.

All ten recorded cases were between fifty-five and seventy-five. All ended disastrously in hospital for suturing and skin grafting. The whirring fan of a 'Dustette' seems a safe six inches inside, but the surgeon remarked, 'They were driven to new lengths by the novelty of the experience.'

Some gentlemen become affectionate towards the doorstep milk bottle, which unlike the real thing is liable to produce penis captivus. As a houseman I encountered a man impassioned of a stone hot-water bottle, the sort then warming beds in Britain's Dickensian country hotels. It was a stonemason's job rather than a surgeon's. As we guardedly chipped away the pottery, the patient commented only that it had seemed a good idea at the time.

124

Ladies have been enamoured of briar pipes, cold-cream jars, the bust of Napoleon, bananas, three oranges (uninspired by Prokofiev). Men of experimental outlook have female vibrators torpedoing up their innards ('the oscillating umbilicus syndrome'). Treatment – let the battery run down.

The resourceful skill, the cheerful unreproach, which medicine applies to mankind's infinite idiosyncracies is illustrated by the book which taught me surgery.

The variety of foreign bodies which have found their way into the rectum is hardly less remarkable than the ingenuity displayed in their removal. A turnip has been delivered per anum by the use of obstetric forceps. A stick firmly impacted has been withdrawn by inserting a gimlet into its lower end. A tumbler, mouth looking downwards, has several times been extracted by filling the interior with a wet plaster of Paris bandage, leaving the end of the bandage extruding, and allowing the plaster to set.

Do not mock the pecadilloes of the old. Only with luck shall we live to enjoy them ourselves.

42

The Reluctant Benefactor
Stillbirth at St Mary's

The discovery of penicillin *a disaster?* It is like complaining the manna was not delivered from Heaven ready sliced.

The invisible penicillin mould did not descend equally miraculously upon Professor Alexander Fleming's poky laboratory in St Mary's Hospital, London. It floated upstairs. The lab below was as thick with moulds as a Neapolitan kitchen with flies. A man was spending his life studying them.

The mould fell upon a small glass plate of nutrient jelly coated with dangerous staphylococcus germs. These would normally be developed in a laboratory incubator like a small oven. Fleming was examining the staphylococci for changes in colour, more obvious if grown in the open air.

It was August 1928. Fleming was off for a month's holiday in his native Scotland. He had finished his experiments, stacked his plates into a bucket of disinfectant. The top plate stood clear of the surface. The mould dropped on the germs at exactly the place and time to attack them. It was a dreadful summer, but the temperature which ruined Fleming's holiday was precisely right for nurturing his penicillin mould.

Back to work, Fleming noticed the forgotten top plate, with a murmur of 'That's funny' examined it, discovered mould to be eating germs. (If you want to see for yourself, the plate is in the British Museum.)

Fleming's discovery thus depended on six successive chances coming up, to an overjoyed punter 'going through the card', a winner on all half-dozen races.

Taciturn, shy, academic Fleming saw penicillin mould as a laboratory tool, gobbling up ubiquitous staphylococci on plates of mixed germs – as from throat swabs – letting more interesting ones grow. Australian Howard Florey at Oxford created *the drug* penicillin. He came across Fleming's research, grew his own mould, refined it and injected it into a patient at the Radcliffe Infirmary, all in eighteen months. Florey had luck, too. His thoughts were illuminated by the discovery of germ killers on Christmas Eve 1932, in Wuppertal. Germany had given the world the first sulpha drug, a month before bestowing upon it Hitler.

Florey made penicillin in milk bottles among the guinea-pig hutches. The Americans made it in brewers' vats. As a minor disaster for Florey, the Americans also patented it and made the money.

There was enough penicillin for the wounded of Eisenhower's and Montgomery's armies by D-day. The disaster was Fleming missing its curative power twelve years earlier. A mitigated one – penicillin was a weapon of war for the Allies, denied to the end the Nazis and Japanese.

43

Rien Ne Va Plus

Disastrous French bedside manner

I often recall to memory an anecdote told by the late Dr Sutherland of Bath. While in Paris, he attended the Hôpital de la Charité. One day he accompanied the physician running through one of the wards to visit the patients, a friar trotting after him with his book in hand to minute down the prescriptions. The doctor stops at a bed, and calls out to the person in it, with the utmost precipitation, Toussez-vous? Suez-vous? Allez vous à la selle? Then turning instantly to the friar, purgez le. Monsieur, il est mort, replied the friar. Diable! Allons! said the doctor, and galloped on with rapidity.

William Cuming (1714–88)

44

The Joy (Slightly Impaired) of Sex

Boswell's clap in 1763

In the autumn of 1762, James Boswell was aged twenty-two, priggish, puritanical, energetic, gregarious, vain, sceptical, witty, superstitious, hypochondriacal, suffering from an anxiety neurosis and dreadfully randy.

He was black-haired, brown-eyed, muddy-complexioned, five foot six and fat. He was the eldest son of a judge, Lord Auchinleck, who lived at Parliament Close near the Court House in Edinburgh, a city of granite morals, vaulted thought, freezing winds and soggy cooking.

Lord Auchinleck was determined James should strut the family path through the law. He educated the youth with tutors, ordinands of the Church of Scotland, young men of impregnable gravity and impeccable bigotry. He sent him to the universities of both Edinburgh and Glasgow.

Lord Auchinleck regarded his son with an eighteenth-century father's natural suspicion. James Boswell attended the theatre, danced attendance on actresses, published boyish verses in the *Scots Magazine*, frivolities to Lord Auchinleck equally despicable. Disinheriting the lad was infuriatingly frustrated by his own marriage contract (his wife Euphemia brought money into the family). He settled for a deed placing James under the control of trustees – chosen by himself – bribing him £100 a year to sign it.

A couple of years before, Boswell had run away to London, two and a half days on horseback, riding round the clock. He hankered to exchange the chilly stone-flagged corridors of Calvinism for the scented gaudy salons of the Roman Catholic Church, which received him at the Bavarian Chapel, Golden Square, Soho. He decided to enter a monastery in France. He met some remarkably jolly fellows and delightfully easygoing girls, and decided against it. After three months, his father demanded he came home.

Lord Auchinleck had one sure, tried way of submitting wayward James to vocational discipline and domestic immobility for life. He would get him married. Boswell took tea with earnestly eligible young ladies in the drawing room, his pleasure with servant girls in the attic. (He fathered a Peggy Doig's child, but gave her £10 to cover costs.) He informed Lord Auchinleck he desired a commission in His Majesty's Footguards. This was not to restore filial probity, but an unchallengeable reason for living permanently in London.

He quit Edinburgh society – as narrow as its wynds, as dull as its weather, as severe as its sermons, as prying as its excisemen's lanterns – at ten in the morning of Monday, 15 November 1762. His chaise rattled down the High Street, the chairmen sagging with sedans seeming to exclaim, 'God prosper long our noble Boswell!' The journey took four days and cost £11.

Boswell stayed in Pall Mall with his friend Andrew Douglas, a Scottish naval surgeon – apprentice-trained, not a bookish member of Henry VIII's Royal College. Boswell dropped joyously into the gossipy, chaffing, tippling, informed, prejudiced, contentious, allusive, humorous male society crowding the scorching fires of London chop houses and coffee houses. But what was an evening's scintillating conversation compared to five delightful minutes with a girl?

Girls were as available as the chops and claret, at the same prices. They paraded the jostling, dung-spattered, lampless Strand north of the Thames, swarmed the Haymarket alongside the Royal Opera House, filled St James's Park under its orderly trees drilled from the Horse Guards to Buckingham House. Boswell took one up an alley off the Strand 'with the intention to enjoy her in armour'. She was at work ill equipped. 'She wondered at my size, and said if I ever took a girl's maidenhead, I would make her squeak. I gave her a shilling, and had enough command of myself to let her go without touching her. I afterwards trembled at the danger I had escaped. I resolved to wait cheerfully till I got some safe girl or was liked by some woman of fashion.'

The armour was either of linen, or a sheep's caecum, the blind end of intestine which extrudes the appendix. The sheep's gut was soaked in alkaline lye, everted, scraped, pickled in burning brimstone, washed with soap, blown up, trimmed to eight inches and threaded at the base with a pretty ribbon for show (officers could order their regimental colours).

The best quality —'Baudruches fines' – were fashioned on oiled moulds, scented with essences, polished with glass rods. The 'Superfine Double' was two caecums gummed together. You bought them from Mrs Phillips at the sign of the Golden Fan and Rising Sun at Orange Court in Leicester Fields, off Piccadilly. Casanova called them English overcoats, and blew them up to send his ladies into fits.

For one sex, they avoided 'the big belly and the squawling brat'. For the other,

> Happy the Man, who in his Pocket keeps,
> Whether with Green or Scarlet Ribband bound,
> A well-made Condom He, nor dreads the Ills
> Of Shankers, or Cordee, or Buboes Dire!

Mrs Douglas talked too much. Boswell moved to Downing Street, forty guineas a year for an upstairs room and use of the parlour all forenoon. The organ which won knowledgeable acclaim remained the tail which wagged the dog. Even in church he laid plans for having women 'from the splendid Madam at fifty guineas a night, down to the civil nymph with white-thread stockings who tramps the Strand', though without disturbing his piety.

In St James's Park with pretty, seventeen-year-old Elizabeth Parker, 'for the first time did I engage in armour, which I found but a dull satisfaction'. (A Yorkshireman once compared it to washing your feet with your boots on.) His open-air harem yielded also an ugly, skinny, sullen girl who stank of gin, and strong, plump, good-humoured Nanny Baker. In our present Prime Minister's garden he enjoyed fresh, agreeable Alice Gibbs – unarmoured, she urged it was so much nicer without and she was as clean as the Queen of England. Fool, fool! he told himself next morning. To have believed one of those abandoned, deceitful wretches! He anticipated the rebuke from Brigadier Mitchner of the Royal Army Medical Corps to World War Two troops – 'Some of you fellows put your private parts where I wouldn't stick the furrule of my umbrella.'

Boswell relished what is technically known as a knee-trembler with a jolly young damsel on Westminster Bridge. He met in the Strand 'a monstrous big whore', took her to a nearby inn where 'she displayed to me all the parts of her enormous carcas', but found her avarice as large as her arse and 'walked off with the gravity of a Barcelonian bishop'. He tried making amends with a little girl up an alley, but could not rise to it.

He almost got a free one from Miss Watts, *grande horizontale* of the Shakespeare tavern, but a paying customer took priority. He collected instead a couple of pretty little girls in Covent Garden, and had them over a bottle of sherry, in order of seniority. On King George III's birthday he dressed in old clothes to spy the night's celebrations, picked up a surly girl in the Park, called himself a barber and settled for sixpence, dangled his linen armour in the Park canal for comfort, had an inconclusive knee-trembler with a wretch in the Strand (sixpence), tried getting it free in Whitehall and reached home at two, much fatigued.

A girl in Whitehall picked his pocket. He had one in the Temple, haunt of lawyers, in the afternoon. A fine fresh lass tapped his shoulder in the Strand, an officer's daughter, born in Gibraltar, irresistible. Then he gloomily left the familiar frolics of London to tour the Continent. Perhaps he consoled himself, tomorrow to fresh whores and pussies new.

Each jig to the carefree music of nightingales brought the vultures of remorse roosting on his morning bedposts. He was revolted at low street debauchery, shocked at intimate union with sluts, determined to do it no more – for twenty-five days at the longest, two at the least. So charming is the frankness of Boswell's frailty. Ours we care not admitting to ourselves, even over bleaker activities like avoiding potatoes.

He longed for a healthy well-bred girl. Amid his boisterous whoring he found one. Her name was Mrs Lewis.

Louisa was an actress. She had played the Queen in *Hamlet*. She was twenty-four, pretty, tall, deep-bosomed, good-natured, vivacious, with 'an enchanting languish in her eyes'. Her husband was Charles Standen, a strolling player who had strolled off. Boswell called for tea. They talked of love, philosophically. He stayed till eight. She hoped he would come again.

He was back next morning. He had woken in a frenzy of love. He declared it bashfully, saying he sought only agreeable conversation and tea. She said he was always welcome. He proclaimed never to contemplate copulation with a woman he did not love. She agreed, adding she was no Platonist. To a man of Boswell's fire, that was a proposition. He kissed her hand and asked how about it? She said, give me time. He mentioned that he was obliged to live with great economy.

He was back after breakfast. She borrowed two guineas off him.

Boswell reckoned the loan a bargain. It would cost more, being cured of something caught from a whore. How about tomorrow? he suggested. She was sick-visiting. Well, the day after? Perhaps. She sang for him.

He arrived two mornings later, exclaimed how neat her lodgings were and threw open the bedroom door to look. She made him sit down and talk of religion. He jumped up, crying, 'You are above the finesse of your sex!' (Be sure always to make a woman better than her sex, he noted that night in his diary.) She asked for more time. *When?* he exclaimed frantically. Friday.

He went home to bread and cheese. It was all he could afford after lending her the two guineas.

On Friday she had second thoughts. He distractedly probed her objections, all as unassailably unsatisfying as any housewife's bedtime headache. He promised in desperation to support any windfall fruit of their union. She told him to cool off for a week.

The week went. He pulled up her petticoats. 'Good heaven, sir!' 'Madam, I cannot help it, I adore you!' She pressed him to her bosom. 'O Mr Boswell!' They fixed on Sunday afternoon, when her landlady was at church.

Wisely not wishing to miss Sunday dinner (roast beef and hot apple pie), Boswell ate an hour early and hurried to Louisa at three. He got the penile equivalent of cold feet. Supposing he was impotent? His anxiety neurosis worsened the probability. She tactfully pretended to forget the agenda of their meeting. He resolutely clutched her alabaster breasts and kissed her delicious lips and led her fluttering into the bedroom. Then her bloody landlady came in. *And* her brother. Boswell cleared out and went to church.

On Monday, Louisa wanted even more time. Tuesday, she fixed Saturday night. She would have Sunday to get over it. Boswell booked at the Black Lion in Water Lane off the Old Bailey, as Mr and Mrs Digges. On Friday, she told him she had started her period.

Ten days of coquettish and physiological frustration ended at eight o'clock on Wednesday night, when Louisa met him in the Piazzas of Covent Garden. A hackney coach waited, with drawn blinds. They arrived at the Black Lion beside Apothecaries Hall, faking the end of a long journey, even to macaroons for munching *en route*.

The couple supped. They drank a few glasses. The maid put on the sheets, well aired. They ordered mulled port floating with fruit for afterwards. Boswell climbed into bed like the challenger climbing into the ring with the champ. He was clasped in her snowy arms and pressed to her milk-white bosom. She was the exquisite mixture of delicacy and wantonness. He did it five times. She said that was three over par. He dozed, fantasizing doing it with other women of his acquaintance. They rose at ten and ate a hearty breakfast. They left by hackney coach and parted in Soho Square.

Five days passed. He felt 'a little heat in the members of my body sacred to Cupid'. Idle fears! He called on Louisa and did it again. Next evening he was out with the boys, to dinner, the play, supper, enormous fun. He got home. 'Too, too plain was Signor Gonorrhoea.'

He was appalled. A dose from a tart was losing a bet in a lively game. From a lady like Louisa, it was like finding yourself mugged in the confessional. 'Those damned twinges, that scalding heat, and that deep-tinged loathsome

133

matter. . . .' His gleet was the blood on Brutus's dagger to dying Caesar. He went to breakfast with Andrew Douglas.

Boswell was familiar with the symptoms. He caught his first dose on the earlier jaunt to London, next year he 'catch'd a Tartar' in Edinburgh. Douglas prescribed confinement to his room, rest, a skimpy diet, aperients and bloodletting. He had hoped for free treatment, but Douglas charged five guineas. Boswell discovered perplexedly, 'The same man as a friend and a surgeon exhibits two very opposite characters.' It was irksome, inhibiting, infuriating. Particularly in scotching his plan shortly to have a go at a Lady Mirabel.

Boswell called on Louisa. He was dignified, bitter, incisive, sorrowful, noble. So would the head of John the Baptist have addressed Salome. She grew pale and atremble. She passionately denied ever having the clap – well, not for fifteen months. He left with icy finality. She falteringly asked if she might continue asking after his health. ' "Madam," said I, archly, "I fancy it will be needless for some weeks." ' He decided she was a most consummate dissembling whore.

Like the syphilitic spirochaete of the Emperor Frederick III, Louisa's gonococcus only slept, to awaken at a lover's caress.

Boswell gave out that he had gone to the country. He suffered bouts of fever so wretched that he glimpsed death. He anguished that his testicle might swell again. He dreamed of Douglas at his bedside pronouncing, 'This is a damned difficult case.' After five weeks, the illness was reduced to a scanty discharge and Douglas freed him. It was a textbook case of untreated gonorrhoea.

An excoriating letter to Louisa demanded his two guineas back. 'If you are not rendered callous by a long course of disguised wickedness, I should think the consideration of your deceit and baseness, your corruption both of body and mind, would be a very severe punishment.' Her servant girl brought a package, unaddressed, without a written word. Boswell relented. Had he been too harsh? He contemplated sending the money back. He decided against it. After all, 'I had come off two guineas better than I expected.'

On 16 May 1763 Boswell met Samuel Johnson. This relationship would have kept many other men's minds off women for life. Not Boswell. He had sixteen more attacks of clap, five illegitimate children and got the crabs in Venice. 'One night of Irish extravagance' in Dublin had him on Kennedy's Lisbon Diet Drink (sasparilla, sasafras, liquorice, guaiac wood, half a guinea a pint). His urinary passages needed irrigation with vitriol, nitrous acid, mercury salts and lead. Ouch. On 31 January 1770 he wrote, 'Earle's: sounded: almost fainted.' The inevitable stricture had developed, to be periodically dilated with metal rods passed up his penis.

On 14 May 1795, Boswell collapsed at a dinner of the Literary Club and was carried home. He could not pass urine. An abscess had developed in his prostate. He died of kidney failure at 2 a.m. on 19 May. At twenty-nine he had married his cousin, who had seven children and three miscarriages.

Boswell's contemporary and counterpart Nicolas Chamfort wrote, *L'amour, tel qui'il existe dans la société, n'est que l'échange de deux fantasies et le contact de deux épidermes.* Love, as it exists in society, is only the exchange of two fantasies and the contact of two epidermises.

It was the only frailty Boswell never confessed. He was too romantic to recognize it.

45

The Joy (Naval Fashion) of Sex
Disastrous effect of shore leave

United States Navy routine, 1913.

In those who have been exposed to infection the entire
penis is scrubbed with liquid soap and water for
several minutes, and then washed with mercuric
perchloride lotion 1:2000. Abrasions are sprayed with
hydrogen peroxide. Two urethral injections of argyrol
(10%) are then given and retained for five minutes.
The whole penis is then rubbed with 33% calomel
ointment which is kept on for several hours.

The Medical Annual

46

One in the Eye
Celebratory disaster

Champagne!
'The only wine which leaves a woman beautiful after
drinking it,' said Madame de Pompadour. Declared Thack-
eray, 'All enjoyments are sensual enjoyments. Shakespeare
and Raphael never invented anything to equal champagne
and oysters, at 5.30 on a hot day.' Robert (Mr Jorrocks)
Surtees mixed it with apricot jam to clean his riding boots.
André Simon's habit of a bottle a day was broken only by
death at ninety-three. 'My God, I am drinking stars!' ex-

claimed Dom Pérignon, who created it at Hautvillers Abbey near Epernay.

Dom Pérignon was the Faraday, the Watt, the Rutherford of oenology. He invented the cork. He got the idea in the summer of 1694, when a pair of Spanish monks arrived with water flasks bunged by cork bark.

The pop of the champagne cork, as exuberant a consort of human joy as laughter itself, has a ghoulish echo of danger.

In swinging 1965, when Britons drank 5,181,185 bottles of champagne, eight Londoners between twenty-four and seventy-two were taken to Moorfields Eye Hospital with injuries from the corks. Seven were serious enough for admission, three developed cataracts. The relevant physics should be in the mind of anyone broaching a bottle of Cliquot.

Chilled champagne (47°F) has an intra-bottle pressure of 90 lb per square inch, rising at room temperature (65°F) and with shaking about. This can shoot the cork 40 feet. (A bottle of claret needs 300 lb force on the corkscrew to open it.) From the formula $V^2 = U^2 + 2fs$ (V = initial U = final velocities in ft/sec, s = distance in feet, f = acceleration of cork in ft/sec) while fiddling with the wire you can calculate that cork strikes eye with a velocity of 45 feet per second. It arrives in half the time of a blink, with a force of 100 atmospheres. This is comparable with blast injuries to the eye in mines and quarries.

To avoid ruining the party, champagne should be opened with a linen napkin over its mouth from the first breaking of the golden foil, the cork eased out pointing at someone else. The Comité Interprofessionel du Vin de Champagne decrees white gloves, but this might be thought *outré* among the canapés. The 'pop' is vulgar. There should be achieved the soft sibilance of an ecstatic sigh from a beautiful woman. Four of the eight patients were waiters, indicating a deplorable sinking of skill since Jeeves.

The injury would never have bothered Dom Pérignon himself. He was blind.

47

Disastrous Disasters

Trop de zèle

At 3 a.m. on 4 February 1976 there was an earthquake in Guatemala. It killed 23,000 and injured 75,000. The world gasped, wrung its hands, poured aid upon the stricken Central Americans.

UNDRO, CARE, CRS and OFDA hit them like inter-continental missiles (United Nations Disaster Relief Organization, Cooperative for American Relief Everywhere, Catholic Relief Service, US Office of Foreign Disaster Assistance). CARE and CRS rushed the Guatemalans 25,000 tons of food. The Guatemalans were not short of food. The local corn lost a third of its price. The local farmers were ruined.

One hundred and fifteen tons of drugs arrived instantly. These included contraceptives, some mysterious tablets made in 1934, tranquillizers, blood-pressure-reducing drugs, and assorted sample packs advertising drugs to American physicians. Three Guatemalan pharmacists tried sorting them out, after three months bulldozed a hole and buried them.

Doctors appeared by the planeload, with prepackaged hospital. None spoke Spanish. The local doctors and nurses were ravenously devouring the work, in a week their hospitals were operating normally. The American hospital was nevertheless erected and treated patients, at £30,000 for each.

There was an earthquake at Lice, Turkey, in 1975. Oxfam hurried 419 polyurethane temporary houses, erected them in sixty days. Two days earlier, the Turkish govern-

ment had finished 1500 permanent relief houses. Everyone
was busy housewarming.

In 1974 the Ethiopian Relief Commission raised the
alarm, if the rains failed again there would be terrible
famine in the south. There was already appalling famine
in the north. Nobody took any notice. A disaster about to
happen is as little news as a dog possibly going to bite a
man. A disaster needs photographs of starving black
babies, howling widows and legless men to make it box
office.

The Ethiopian famine arrived as promised. The United
Nations created camps to feed the nomadic victims, and
killed many of them with diseases to which their isolated
life left them susceptible.

People do not all panic, go mad, flee like lemmings after
disasters. Not all disasters bring horrific epidemics, despite
photographs of cleanly white doctors and nurses painfully
sticking needles into everyone in sight. All disaster-struck
governments are not corrupt. Food may be scattered but
not destroyed. Nobody loses all their clothes or all their
friends. 'Experts have not been able to trace a single recorded death from exposure after disaster,' the *Sunday Times*
reported, 'even in extremely cold conditions.'

When up against raw Nature, man intelligently impro-
vises. Otherwise, he would never have evolved to enjoy the
comforts which competing relief agencies hustle so hap-
hazardly to restore.

48

The Final Diagnosis

Still dodgy

A Welsh GP:

> Why don't you say it? Of course he's dead. But you
> must be sure. Once said it can't be unsaid. . . . It
> leaves you with an uneasy feeling that after half an
> hour in the Chapel of Rest the patient will sit up and
> ask for a large Scotch without ice.

At noon on 21 November 1741, Jane Brown, delirious
with smallpox, threw herself into the New River at Islington in north London. She was noticed floating face down
by an old man on the opposite bank, who tottered to raise
the alarm at the Crown alehouse, some way off.

The only problem for the citizens who dragged her out
was the right parish to bury her – Islington or next door
Clerkenwell. After a wrangle, they had Bill Stevens the
gravedigger and Tom Bull the parish bearer carry the
corpse to Clerkenwell's St James's workhouse. It was
frosty. Bill slipped on the grass. The body fell. Restoring
it to their shoulders, they heard a groan.

The workhouse master was unimpressed. He laid Jane
on the lid of the parish coffin in the cold outside the infirmary door, ordained spot for inmates awaiting burial. A
human body is always an object of interest. A passer-by
noticed her upper lip quiver. They put her to bed and sent
for Mr Osborne, surgeon and apothecary.

It was then three in the afternoon. He found her cold,
pulseless, distended. He effected urgent resuscitation with
spirit of hartshorn in warm water. They rubbed her with
coarse cloths. She croaked. She belched. Up came the river
water. They tipped her head down, it ran everywhere.

Mr Osborne next administered the sliced ginger in mountain wine, but she seemed to have died again. He sent urgently for the hot flannel petticoat. Jane's jaw trembled, she rumbled, belched mightily, moved an arm. More ginger and wine. Her pulse fluttered. They wrapped her all over in warm flannel, the emergency medicines arrived, they gave her Raleigh's confection and tincture of cardamom. At eight, she was supping off broth and bread.

Next morning Jane felt splendid, if sore all over. In a week she was walking round the ward, complaining only of everlasting hunger. Her smallpox got better, too.

In 1773, Patrick Redmond, condemned for robbery, was hanged on the Irish gallows for twenty-nine minutes by the stopwatch. He was cut down, hastened by friends to nearby fields as the sheriff retired, given a tobacco clyster and stimulated with lighted pipes. The mob rubbed his limbs in relays from two in the afternoon until six, when his neck encouragingly began to bleed. The sheriff heard of the insolent wake, the mob whisked their patient from under his nose, kept him two days on warm brandy and water lying on stable hay, sped him off to avoid capture. Patrick was later said to be fine in County Clare.

A Swedish gardener in 1676, upright for sixteen hours in sixty feet of freezing water at Tronningholm, was restored to life by heat from the stove. The Russians were always suffocating themselves from stoves, but revived when rolled in the snow. When Ann Green was hanged at Oxford in 1650, her corpse was handled so roughly it woke her up. Doctors think she had an ossified larynx.

The bell gloomily tolls for all mankind, the messenger galloping up as the firing squad cocks its rifles cheerfully reprieves us all.

But even Lazarus died sometime.

49

Greatest Disaster of All

Pressing proclivity to procreate

The world population increases by one million every Monday to Friday.

It took from cavemen to 1830 to reach 1000 million, from the crinoline to the Charleston to reach 2000 million, from Hitler to Krushchev to reach 3000 million, from the Beatles to Mrs Thatcher to reach 4000 million.

By 2112 it will level out at 10,500 million, two and a half times what it is now. Or perhaps at 14,200 million in 2132, the United Nations is not sure. Though with luck, we might be only 8000 million in 2040. The roads will still be dreadfully busy.

The increase will be lopsided. In 2110, the rich countries will be only 13 per cent of the global population, against 24 per cent today. Europe will stop increasing itself by 2030, and American in 2060. The Third World will then have tripled itself, to 9100 million.

'While imbalances created by poverty, malnutrition or ill health persist,' say the United Nations, 'the social tensions arising out of population pressures will permeate every aspect of life on earth.'

Luckily, we are steadily killing ourselves and hardly noticing it.

'As much as 50 per cent of mortality from the ten leading causes of death in the United States can be traced to lifestyle,' says the US National Institute of Medicine. Threequarters of Americans die from heart and circulatory disease, cancer, accidents or violence, which they bring upon themselves with cigarettes (one-third of Americans over nineteen smoke), alcohol (134 million drink, often too much), drugs, driving, quack medicines and 'maladaptive responses to social pressures'.

The rich nations *must* respond to idealistic urgings and help the poor ones. Once the benefits of civilization come to Africa and Southern Asia, they will kill themselves off just as eagerly.

50

Disastrous End

Man's activities have been hopelessly open to disaster since that calamitous business of the serpent in the Garden of Eden. Best treatment is to admit, to analyse, to avoid. Medicine readily confesses its share. But what a disaster, were there no doctors amid the world's unending catalogue of disasters.

> The profession of medicine and surgery must always rank as the most noble that man can adopt. The spectacle of a doctor in action among soldiers (or sailors) in equal danger with equal courage, saving life where all others are taking it, allaying pain where all others are causing it, is one which must always seem glorious, whether to God or man.

The writer brought us through the greatest disaster of this century.

Thank you, Sir Winston.

If you can meet with Triumph and Disaster
And treat those two impostors just the same . . .

Rudyard Kipling

Acknowledgements

To the Wellcome Institute for the History of Medicine, the library of the Royal College of Surgeons of England and the London Library.

To the Editor of *Punch*, for kind permission to reproduce the verse in Chapter 26, Doctor Death.

To A. D. Peters & Co. Ltd for kind permission to reproduce Pepys' Diary in Chapter 27, And so to Bed.

References

1 Triple Knock-Out
Flemming, P. Robert Liston, the first professor of clinical surgery at UCH. *University College Hospital Magazine*, 1926. **1**:176–85.
Cock, W. F. The first operation under ether in Europe. *University College Hospital Magazine*, 1911. **1**: *127–44*.

2 Untreasured Island
Sunday Times, 19 April 1981.
The Times, 25 May 1981.

3 Transatlantic Disaster
Garrison, E. H. *History of medicine* (4th edn). Philadelphia: Saunders, 1929: 189–92.
Guthrie, D. *A history of medicine* (2nd edn). London: Nelson, 1958: 164–5.

4 Ironing Out the Bugs in Panama
Scott, H. H. *A history of tropical medicine*. London: Arnold, 1939.

5 Surgical Souvenirs
The Medical Defence Union annual report, 1980: 20.

6 The Green Monkeys
Vella, E. E. Marburg virus disease. *Update*, January 1977.
Trials of war criminals before the Nuremberg Military Tribunals under Control Council Law No. 10 (vii) Washington, 1952. Trial of Professor Hörlein: 245.

7 A Touch of Class
Garrison, F. H. *History of medicine* (4th edn). Philadelphia: Saunders, 1929: 288.

8 Boob Boobs
Daily Telegraph, 6 June 1979.

9 Rude Awakening
The Medical Defence Union annual report, 1980: 55.

10 Typhoid Mary
Kellock, I. A. The curious career of 'Typhoid Mary'.
Manchester University Medical School Gazette, 1955. **34**:
133–6.
Strange fever. *MD*, 1969. **13**: 220–6.

11 Disastrous Motherhood
Holmes, O. W. On the contagiousness of puerperal fever.
New England Quarterly Journal of Medicine, Boston (1842–3).
i: 503–30.

13 Scurvy Treatment
Orwell, G. *The road to Wigan Pier*. London: Gollancz, 1937.
Cyriax, R. J. *Sir John Franklin's last Arctic expedition*. London:
Methuen, 1939.
Drummond, J. C., and Wilbraham, A. *The Englishman's food*
(2nd edn). London: Cape, 1957.

14 The Emperor's Sore Throat
Stevenson, R. S. *Morell Mackenzie*. London: Heinemann,
1946.
Holland, C. *The notebooks of a spinster lady 1878–1903*.
London: Cassell, 1919: 268.
Financial Times, 23 January 1982.

15 The Tender Trap
Chatelaine, April 1976.

17 The Most Unkindest Cut of All
Walsham, W. J. and Spencer, W. G. *Surgery, its theory and
practice* (8th edn). London: Churchill, 1903: 1005.
Delvin, D. Blackballed. *World Medicine*, 28 June 1978:
134–6.
Vessey, M., Lawless, M., and Yeates, D. Efficacy of
different contraceptive methods. *Lancet*, 1982. i:841–2.

18 Bitter Victory
Beveridge, W. I. B. *Influenza, the last great plague*. London:
Heinemann, 1977: 30–33, 40–44.
Osborn, J. E. *History, science and politics. Influenza in America
1918–1976*. New York: Prodist, 1977; 4–13.

Hoehling, A. A. *The great epidemic*. Boston: Little Brown, 1961:77.

Katz, R. S. Flu 1918–19: a further study in mortality. *Bulletin of the History of Medicine*, 1977, **51**:617–19.

19 St Anthony's Fire

Gabbai, Lisbonne, Pourquier. Ergot poisoning at Pont St Esprit. *British Medical Journal*, 1951. ii:650–51.

British Medical Journal, 1951.ii:596.

Brown, P. W. F. Bread poisoning. *Notes & Queries*, 1957. **4**:6–7.

Van Zwanenberg, D. A 'singular calamity'. *Medical History*, 1973.**17**:204–7.

Caporael, L. R. Ergotism: the Satan loosed in Salem? *Science*, 1976, **192**:21–6.

Spanos, N. P. and Gottlieb, J. Ergotism and the Salem village witch trials. *Science*, 1976. **194**:1390–94.

20 Beachy Head

Surtees, S. J. Suicide and accidental death at Beachy Head. *British Medicial Journal*, 1982:i.321–4.

The Times, 29 May 1982.

Irvine, M. What causes death? *World Medicine*, 9 January 1982.

21 The King is Dead

British Medical Journal, 1910. i:1557–60.

Guthrie, D. *A history of medicine* (2nd edn). London: Nelson, 1958.

Miller, J. *The body in question*. London: Cape, 1978.

Latham, R. and Matthews, W. (eds.). *The diary of Samuel Pepys* (iv). London: Bell, 1971.

22 Obstetrical Obsession

The Times, 25 September 1981.

23 Sandwich Disaster

British Medical Journal, 1922. ii:394, 481, 527–8.

The Times, 18, 19, 21, 23, 25, 26 August, 5, 6, 7, 8 September 1922.

24 Breaking It Off

Johnson, G. R. and Corriere, J. N. Partial priapism. *Journal of Urology*, 1980. **124**:147.

25 101 Uses of a Dead Pope
Daily Telegraph, 14 May 1981.

26 Doctor Death
Dictionary of National Biography 1941–1950.
Browne, D. G., and Tullett, E. V. *Bernard Spilsbury*.
  London: Harrap, 1951.
Orwell, G. *Decline of the English murder*. Harmondsworth:
  Penguin, 1965.
Punch, 1928. **174**:305.

27 And so to Bed
Latham, R., and Matthews, W. (eds.). *The diary of Samuel
  Pepys* (ix). London: Bell, 1976.

28 Luckless Lübeck
Trollope, A. *An autobiography*. Edinburgh & London,
  Blackwood, 1883.
Dubois, R. and J. *The white plague*. London: Gollancz, 1953.
Irvine, K. N. *BCG vaccination in theory and practice*. Oxford:
  Blackwell, 1949.

29 The Decline and Fall of Edward Gibbon
Gibbon, E. *Autobiography*. Oxford: University Press, 1907.
Dale, P. M. *Medical Biographies*. Norman: University of
  Oklahoma Press, 1952:112–17.

30 The Sack-'em-Up Men
Guthrie, D. *A history of medicine* (2nd edn). London: Nelson,
  1958.
Roughhead, W. *Burke and Hare* (trial). Edinburgh: Hodge,
  1921.
Walbrook, H. M. *Murders and murder trials 1812–1912*.
  London: Constable, 1932.

31 A Lousy Trick
Garrison, F. H. *History of medicine* (4th edn), Philadelphia:
  Saunders, 1929: 242–3.

32 The Black Death
Ziegler, P. *The Black Death*. London: Collins, 1969.

33 Everyday Disaster
Financial Times, 5 September 1981

References

Bowsher, W. G., and Kenyon, G. S. Accidental
oropharyngeal injury. *British Medical Journal*, 1982. i:1751–2.
Daneshmend, T. K., and Campbell, M. J. Dark Warrior
epilepsy. *British Medical Journal*, 1982, i:1751–2.
The Times, 16 April; 16, 17, September, 1981.

34 Love Locked In
Taylor, E. K. Penis captivus – did it occur? *British Medical
Journal*, 1979. ii:977–8.

35 Suffer the Little Children
Baker, I. A., *et al.* School milk and growth in primary
schoolchildren. *Lancet*, 1978. ii:575.
Sunday Times, 10 September 1978.
The Times, 2 September; 1 October 1981.

36 Kinky Kinks
Shaw, G. B. *The doctor's dilemma*. 1906.
Layton, T. B. *Sir William Arbuthnot Lane, Bart*, Edinburgh:
Livingstone, 1956.

37 The Dying Art
Smith, S. *Forensic medicine* (8th edn). London: Churchill,
1945:258.
Duff, C. *A handbook on hanging*. London: Cayme Press, 1928.
Maugham, W. S. *A writer's notebook*. London: Heinemann,
1949:254.
Healey, T. The good Dr Guillotin and his humane
machine. *World Medicine*, 5 April 1978:61–71.
Weiner, D. B. The real Doctor Guillotin. *Journal of the
American Medical Association*, 1972. **220**:85–9.
Soubiran, A. *The Good Doctor Guillotin*. London: Souvenir
Press, 1964:167.

38 Clubland Doctor
Griffith, E. F. *Doctors by themselves*. London: Cassell, 1951:
63.

39 Design for Living
Woodham-Smith, C. *Florence Nightingale*. Harmondsworth:
Penguin, 1955.
The Times, 23 January, 18 March 1982.
Sunday Times, 31 January 1982.

40 Terror in the Tucker

Murphy, K. J. Bilateral renal calculi and aminoaciduria after excessive intake of Worcestershire sauce. *Lancet,* 1967. ii:401–2.

Hornadge, B. (ed.). *The ugly Australian.* Sydney: Bacchus Books, 1976:118, 124.

41 Cleaner Living

Fox, M., and Barrett E. L. 'Vacuum cleaner injury' of the penis. *British Medical Journal,* 1960. ii:1942.

Citron, N. D., and Wade, P. J. Penile injuries from vacuum cleaners. *British Medical Journal,* 1980: ii:26.

Zufall, R. Laceration of the penis from hand vacuum cleaners. *Journal of the American Medical Association* 1973. **224**:630.

Bailey, H., and Love, R. J. M. *A short practice of surgery* (6th edn). London: Lewis, 1943: 399.

43 Rien Ne Va Plus

Griffith, E. F. *Doctors by themselves.* London: Cassell, 1951: 68.

44 The Joy (Slightly Impaired) of Sex

Pottle, A. F. (ed.). *Boswell's London journal 1762–1763.* London: Heinemann, 1950.

Ober, W. B. *Boswell's clap and other essays.* Carbondale & Edwardsville: South Illinois University Press, 1979.

Freyer, P. *The birth controllers.* London: Secker & Warburg, 1965.

45 The Joy (Naval Fashion) of Sex

World Medicine 30 May 1981, 58.

46 One in the Eye

Archer, D., and Galloway, N. Champagne-cork injury to the eye. *Lancet.* 1967, ii:487–9.

47 Disastrous Disasters

Sloan, S. Just another disaster. *World Medicine,* 11 January 1978.

Sunday Times, 25 June 1978.

48 The Final Diagnosis

Humphreys, R. Diagnosing death. *World Medicine,* 14 June 1980: 55.

References

Wood, S. Resuscitation in 1741. *British Medical Journal*, 1951. ii:671.

Schuster, N. H. The Emperor of Russia and the Royal Humane Society. *Journal of the Royal College of General Practitioners*, 1971. **21**:634.

Payne, J. P. On the resuscitation of the apparently dead. *Annals of the Royal College of Surgeons of England*, 1964. **45**:98.

49 Greatest Disaster of All
The Times, 17 June 1981; 10 July 1982.

50 Disastrous End
Roddis, L. H. *James Lind*. New York: Schuman, 1950:3.